Fasting for Life wisely and convincingly shows us how disciplined fasting encourages physical, mental, and spiritual well-being. A PhD-trained chemist and a committed Christian, Dr. Umesiri draws upon his scientific training and his spiritual insight to help the "lay" reader see the holistic benefits of fasting. It is a fascinating and convicting book that gracefully calls us to discipline our appetite for food as we deepen our longing for God.

—Dr. Charles W. Pollard
President, John Brown University

Fasting for Life

Fasting for Life

Francis E. Umesiri, PhD

SILOAM

Most CHARISMA HOUSE BOOK GROUP products are available at special quantity discounts for bulk purchase for sales promotions, premiums, fund-raising, and educational needs. For details, write Charisma House Book Group, 600 Rinehart Road, Lake Mary, Florida 32746, or telephone (407) 333-0600.

FASTING FOR LIFE by Francis E. Umesiri, PhD
Published by Siloam
Charisma Media/Charisma House Book Group
600 Rinehart Road
Lake Mary, Florida 32746
www.charismahouse.com

Cover design by Vincent Pirozzi
Design Director: Justin Evans

Visit the author's website at www.francisumesiri.com.

Library of Congress Cataloging-in-Publication Data:
Names: Umesiri, Francis E., author.
Title: Fasting for life / Francis E. Umesiri.
Description: First edition. | Lake Mary, Florida : Siloam, [2015]
Identifiers: LCCN 2015036225| ISBN 9781629986265 (paperback) | ISBN
    9781629986272 (e-book)
Subjects: LCSH: Fasting--Therapeutic use. | Fasting--Spiritual aspects.
Classification: LCC RM226 .U44 2015 | DDC 613.2/5--dc23
LC record available at http://lccn.loc.gov/2015036225

This book contains the opinions and ideas of its author. It is solely for informational and educational purposes and should not be regarded as a substitute for professional medical treatment. The nature of your body's health condition is complex and unique. Therefore, you should consult a health professional before you begin any new exercise, nutrition, or supplementation program or if you have questions about your health. Neither the author nor the publisher shall be liable or responsible for any loss or damage allegedly arising from any information or suggestion in this book.

While the author has made every effort to provide accurate Internet addresses at the time of publication, neither the publisher nor the author assumes any responsibility for errors or for changes that occur after publication.

First edition

16 17 18 19 20 — 987654321
Printed in the United States of America

*Dedicated to my wife (Toyin), our
two sons (Isaac and David), and
the precious little one on the way.
You all mean the world to me.*

CONTENTS

Part 1

The Science of Fasting

Part 2

Fasting for the Whole Person

ACKNOWLEDGMENTS

I AM THANKFUL FOR THE MANY AUTHORS WHOSE writings have helped to shape the thoughts and style reflected in my own writings. In particular I acknowledge the influence that Eugene Peterson's writings have had on my Christian walk—especially with regards to my constant desire to embrace what God is doing right now in the place and time where I am located.

I am also thankful to Pastor and Mrs. Sam Adelusimo and the members of Chapel of Praise Northwest Arkansas for their total support and embrace of the message of fasting.

Many thanks to Jevon Bolden, former senior acquisitions editor at Charisma House. She took a chance on the book and spent a lot of time editing and correcting it.

FOREWORD

THE WORLD OFTEN WONDERS AT THE POSSIBILITY OF integration between science and faith. But history gives us enough examples of great thinkers and scientists whose works were directly or indirectly impacted by their faith. A few examples will suffice: from Newton (gravity); Pascal, who based a lot of his thinking on Pascal's law (physics), Pascal's theorem (math), and Pascal's wager (theology) on the Scriptures; Carolus Linnaeus, who used the Scriptures as a basis to develop the nomenclature for naming plants and animals; to modern-day individuals such as Sir Robert Boyd, former president of Royal Astronomical Society, and Nobel laureate in chemistry Richard Smalley (1996 Nobel Prize Chemistry). Professor Umesiri, through this book, is taking a cue from such historical precedence to effectively show that science often supports and affirms the things that the Lord teaches the church.

Umesiri, the scientist, has taken on a little appreciated but deeply needed spiritual discipline of fasting. Jesus made it clear that fasting is the basis for victory over evil and that without it signs and wonders are impossible. Umesiri, the man of faith, has shown the world the practicality of fasting as a critical tool for optimizing bodily functions. In carrying out this great task, Professor Umesiri has caused, "Physical training is good, but training for godliness is much better, promising benefits in this life and in the life to come" (1 Tim. 4:8, NLT) to come alive.

I am particularly intrigued by his engagement with understanding of brain health and freedom from diabetes, cancer, and cardiovascular diseases. Do these diseases qualify as the modern-day manifestation of that which will *not* go away without fasting and prayers? Is there a correlation between consistent commitment to the spiritual discipline of fasting and a freedom from the "diseases of Egypt"? Although we are yet to scientifically prove a direct linkage between these diseases and the demoniac elements, Professor Umesiri has scientifically proven that we can be free from their impact through fasting.

I heartily recommend this book for its practicality, its deep spirituality, and its true integrational intent—it is showing us again that science and God are *not* contraindicative!

—JAMES O. FADEL
SPECIAL ASSISTANT TO GENERAL OVERSEER AND CHAIRMAN
THE REDEEMED CHRISTIAN CHURCH OF GOD,
NORTH AMERICA

Part 1

THE SCIENCE OF FASTING

Chapter 1

WHY FASTING MATTERS

The doctor of the future will give no medication, but will
interest his patients in the care of the human frame,
diet, and in the cause and prevention of disease.

—FAMED INVENTOR THOMAS EDISON[1]

A S A MEDICINAL CHEMIST, COLLEGE PROFESSOR,
and medical writer, I am not only passionate about
the field of scientific discovery, but also about
communicating key discoveries that will benefit the public.
This is even truer when a particular scientific finding
appears to validate centuries-old spiritual disciplines. I
write this book, therefore, with a sense of responsibility:
a responsibility to share with you interesting biomedical
discoveries that—if you act on them—can literally reduce
your risk of falling victim to various chronic diseases.

Several years ago I read a fascinating article in the
leading journal *Science*. It referenced ongoing research

in the area of fasting (what scientists call "caloric restriction" or "intermittent fasting"). The findings immediately caught my attention. Although in the past I had fasted regularly for many years, I gradually had stopped. Like most Americans, I found it harder to skip a meal or two in order to focus on God. Now, jolted by news of the promising prospects of fasting, I initiated a thorough review of scientific research covering the previous seven decades. I reviewed a number of original and peer-reviewed articles published in highly regarded journals. The sheer volume of credible research pointing to the immense health benefits of fasting—meaning sustained reduction in energy intake—overwhelmed me. The results staring me in the face forced me to change my habits. Returning to my roots, I resumed intermittent fasting.

Next, the medical writer in me took over. I wondered why so many people seemed unaware of these studies. I came away convinced that now is the time to help the public become aware of fasting's health benefits. In this book I will share basic facts about these benefits, as documented in highly reputable, peer-reviewed journals (peer-reviewed literature being the gold standard for scientific and academic writings). Some of those studies were funded by the National Institute on Aging, an arm of the National Institutes of Health (NIH).

What you will read in the pages that follow are pure scientific facts. No hype. No exaggerations. This is not a faddish diet or weight-loss program. I am a medicinal chemist, not a dietician. I am confident that, given the raw scientific facts in reasonably understandable language, people will make up their own minds and apply such facts accordingly. Studies in this area are still ongoing. Still, almost every bit of credible research on animal models (from rats to monkeys), as well as humans, has shown a significant improvement in the ability of fasting to reduce the risk of such major diseases as cancer, diabetes, stroke, and cardiovascular and neurodegenerative diseases—in some cases, by reductions of up to 50 percent.

I have chosen to highlight relatively few articles while still demonstrating the scientific proof of fasting's benefits. Instead of an exhaustive list, these highlighted articles are only representative of the vast scope of material published on this topic.

My hope is that this book will serve as a catalyst and spur you to action. After all, heart attack, diabetes, cancer, stroke, and Alzheimer's disease represent serious, deadly diseases. Their presence has grown to such alarming proportions in the Western world that it demands we take all the preventive efforts we can muster.

The big three

Let's look at three of the aforementioned diseases: diabetes, heart disease, and cancer.

- Diabetes is a huge problem—so huge that no one should take it for granted.

According to a recent Centers for Disease Control and Prevention report on diabetes, 9.3 percent of Americans (29.1 million persons) are affected by diabetes.[2] Diabetes is the leading cause of kidney failure, nontraumatic lower limb amputations, and new cases of blindness among adults in the United States. Also a major cause of heart disease and stroke, diabetes is the seventh-leading cause of death in the nation. There is a tendency to read such statistics and simply wave your hand, guessing it somehow will not strike you. While I wish that everyone reading these words would not be affected by the devastating effects of this disease, it is important that each person take preventive steps to avoid contracting it. Fasting can definitely help.

- Cardiovascular (heart) diseases are the leading killer in the United States.

The World Health Organization (WHO) affirms that heart disease and associated cardiovascular diseases (CVDs) are the number one cause of death both in this country and across the world. About 17.5 million people died from CVDs in 2012, representing 31 percent of all global deaths. Of these deaths, an estimated 7.4 million were due to coronary heart disease and 6.7 million were due to stroke.[3] The WHO projects that by the year 2030, the number of people who die annually from CVDs will surpass 23 million. The good news is that you can reduce your risk for this killer disease through fasting. It is such an encouraging, and yet simple, prescription that I feel a sense of duty to share some of the ongoing scientific results. While fasting is not a "cure all" panacea, it can provide significant benefits in the fight against heart disease.

- Cancer is the second-worst killer, one you must avoid at all costs.

The American Cancer Society estimated that in 2015, more than 1.6 million new cancer cases would be diagnosed, with more than 589,000 Americans projected to die from cancer, or more than 1,600 people per day.[4] One of every four deaths in the United States is a result of some form of cancer. While there is no "bulletproof" method for preventing cancer, studies strongly suggest that fasting can significantly reduce one's risks of contracting this disease. Considering how ravaging this disease can be, any meaningful steps to prevent or reduce the risks are certainly worth trying.

As a result of the far-reaching nature of these diseases, I will focus on discussing some of the health benefits of fasting in relation to the major chronic diseases: diabetes, coronary heart failure, stroke, memory loss (including Alzheimer's disease), and cancer. It is my hope that you study this material with an open mind; consult the publications referenced here as a starting point to further investigate this for yourself.

If these health benefits represented all there is to fasting, they would still be amazing. However, as a Christian who understands the spiritual implications of fasting, these studies made it all the more imperative for me to take this subject seriously. Fasting has tremendous benefits to the soul, a fact all major religions have long acknowledged (and practiced). To get the maximum benefits from fasting, I suggest that you approach it from a holistic view—spirit, soul, and body. Because of this, I included a section on fasting as a spiritual discipline and from a Christian perspective. The Bible has a lot to say about fasting and its possible role in spiritual renewal.

Chapter 2

WHEN LESS IS MORE

The public in industrialized countries is bombarded with a bewildering array of information on the effects of dietary factors on health. However, the only well-established means of improving health through diet is maintaining a relatively low caloric intake.

—MARK MATTSON, CHIEF OF THE LABORATORY OF
NEUROSCIENCES AT THE NATIONAL INSTITUTE ON AGING[1]

THERE IS CREDIBLE BIOMEDICAL EVIDENCE THAT fasting improves health span, both in animal and human studies. This is what inspired me to distill some of this evidence and provide easily understood explanations of how fasting can improve your health, including your health span. Calorie restriction (CR) or fasting delays the development of age-associated diseases and increases health span in rodents, monkeys, and humans.

What is health span? Simply put, it is the time of life in which we are free from disposition to disease. A strong health span reflects an increased quality of life and prolonged health during our senior years. Radically different from life span, health span involves prolonged delay in the onset of age-associated diseases. While we all want to live to an old age, we want that to be a healthy, disease-free existence. While research on short-lived animals has conclusively shown that fasting can and does prolong life span, studies on humans are ongoing and seek to ascertain whether calorie restriction can also increase human life span. Still, most scientific studies involving primates and human beings reveal this: *in virtually all studies fasting improves almost all indicators of good health measured in humans.*

As I said in chapter 1, fasting can significantly reduce your risk of cancer, stroke, diabetes, and such neurodegenerative diseases as Parkinson's and Alzheimer's. I haven't included any statements that aren't substantiated by more than seventy years of biomedical research. Studies on animal models have already conclusively proven the improvements on those species' health span. And while researchers need to conduct more randomized, clinical trials involving large numbers of subjects, I will show that several studies involving humans have revealed that fasting consistently reduces health risk markers across the spectrum. In fact, while reviewing available scientific support for fasting to improve brain health, physicians from the National Institute on Aging's Intramural Research Program had this to say:

> We are now at a stage where our knowledge of both the genetic and environmental factors which have been linked to unsuccessful brain aging, and their cellular and molecular consequences, can be

utilized to provide the general population with advice on aging successfully. In this review, we will discuss two dietary strategies, caloric restriction and intermittent fasting, which could potentially be used to mediate successful aging and forestall the onset of certain neurodegenerative disorders.[2]

Increased health span

This book is doing exactly what these doctors and others are advocating: utilizing the vast body of current scientific evidence in support of fasting to provide the general public with advice on successful aging and increasing their health span. Still, before one can dispense such pertinent advice, it will be helpful to call our attention directly to the body of scientific proof that strongly supports the idea of fasting's benefits.

Many in the scientific community tend to assume that popular culture does not have either the appetite or the capacity to understand scientific facts. This assumption is wrong for two reasons:

- First, it tends to underestimate the ability of individuals to seek out information or change when motivated to do so.

What could offer more motivation than living a healthy life and avoiding early onset of chronic, debilitating diseases? Other dreams and aspirations of life tend to hang on this health factor. I am betting on the idea that you are rational enough—and motivated enough for self-survival—to be willing to spend a few hours assimilating information that could literally alter the trajectory of your health.

- The other false assumption about the general populace is its capacity, or lack thereof, to absorb scientific facts.

Could it be that scientists have been rather guilty of using too much jargon and parochial language in describing their findings to be of help to any person (including other scientists) who doesn't earn a living from that particular discipline? Now, it is true that the nature of scientific inquiry, and the specificity required, lend themselves to specialty-specific language. Yet it seems almost an understatement that science can do a better job of communicating its findings to those not directly involved in that area of research. I am convinced that our friends and family members are capable and willing to digest relevant scientific information—that is, when it is written in the same kind of language they use for day-to-day communication.

Therefore, I set out within these pages to perform the delicate dance between describing the most up-to-date scientific findings regarding fasting and health and using language that anyone on the street can understand and appreciate. While this is possible, it is certainly not an easy undertaking. It underscores why most scientists tend to leave this task alone. As a scientist, educator, and medical writer, I hope to utilize my experience and training to bridge the gap between science and people who may need its findings.

Why eating less is healthy

In a study published by the National Institutes of Health, the authors wrote: "Put simply, high energy intake increases, while low energy intake decreases, the risks of cardiovascular disease, type 2 diabetes, stroke, cancers and possibly neurodegenerative disorders."[3] Some scientists speculate that perhaps the reason certain regions of the world where people eat much less (either due to lack or cultural and religious considerations) seem to have less incidence of cancer, stroke, and other diseases may be due in part to the hormetic effect of calorie reduction.

Inversely is it possible that the high prevalence of diseases associated with developed and industrialized nations stems—at least in part—from our overindulgence in food? Many scientists involved in healthy aging, nutritional studies, and physiology seem to think so. For example, after reviewing studies involving hormetic effects of fasting, a researcher with the NIH concluded: "The public in industrialized countries is bombarded with a bewildering array of information on the effects of dietary factors on health. However, the only well-established means of improving health through diet is maintaining a relatively low caloric intake."[4]

In chapter 4 I discuss the role of hormesis in relation to fasting in some detail. But suffice it to note at this point that the theory of hormetic effect suggests that repeated exposure to mild stress (which includes fasting, among others) increases resistance of cells to other forms of disease pathways.

There are five main determinants of health used by medical and health practitioners around the world to gauge or guide the health-care system:

- Genetic disposition—because of their parentage, certain people have predispositions to certain diseases.

- Social circumstances—people with lower socioeconomic status tend to die earlier and have more disabilities.

- Environmental exposure—this includes exposure to such toxic materials as lead paint, polluted air and water, dangerous neighborhoods, and lack of outlets for physical activity.

- Behavioral patterns—this includes obesity, inactivity, tobacco or alcohol use, and drug intake.

- Health-care access—namely, doctor visits and inpatient or outpatient treatment and care.

It may surprise you to know that of all these five health determinants, the biggest contributor to premature death in the United States is behavioral patterns. Dr. Steven A. Schroeder spelled this out in an article published in the *New England Journal of Medicine* titled, "We Can Do Better—Improving the Health of the American People." He spelled out how behavior contributes to a whopping 40 percent of all preventable diseases in this country.

Meanwhile, health care contributes only 10 percent.[5] In other words, out of every one hundred persons who die prematurely (before reaching good old age) in this country, forty of them could have lived if they had changed their behavior as it relates to their health. Only ten of those deaths were a result of an inability to get the right, or adequate, health care.

High cost of health care

Given these statistics, I find it quite surprising that health care takes an overwhelming chunk of the money allocated to health. In 2006 alone the United States spent a whopping $2.1 trillion on health care, which accounted for 16 percent of the nation's gross domestic product.[6] Most professionals in the health field agree that the health-care system, as currently structured, is probably not equipped to handle behavioral determinants. Many doctors do their best to help patients embrace changes in their lifestyle. However, it is also widely accepted that behavioral factors may be beyond the scope of traditional medical training programs, even if only in terms of their focus.

Sadly, what this means is that there is little or nothing your medical doctor can do about a major determinant of your health. Health care is different from health. A doctor's training prepares him well enough to solve your health *problems* rather than address *prevention*. Fortunately current efforts in preventive medicine are gaining more ground. As such, more and more doctors are going out of their way to venture into behavioral issues in order to help their patients. But beyond that, there is not much more a doctor can do for you when it comes to living in good health, aging successfully, and delaying the early onset of age-associated diseases.

To boil it down to a simple fact, your health is your responsibility. Dr. Schroeder's article also pointed out that obesity and corresponding inactivity, and smoking account for a much larger percentage of preventable deaths in the United States—all behavioral choices. When Schroeder's article appeared in 2007, more than 435,000 persons died from smoking, a figure that has since risen above 440,000. Another 365,000 individuals died from obesity- and inactivity-related complications.[7] Considering the preventable nature of these sad statistics, it seems a tad astonishing that these aspects of our nation's health appear to receive significantly less attention and money than matters dealing with health care.

In fact, in his discussion of smoking, Dr. Schroeder writes: "Given the effects of smoking on health, the relative inattention to tobacco by those federal and state agencies charged with protecting the public health is baffling and disappointing."[8] And he concludes: "The single greatest opportunity to improve health and reduce premature deaths lies in personal behavior."[9]

It is this "single greatest opportunity to improve health" that I am focusing on; in other words, how we can benefit from fasting and intentionally reducing our caloric intake.

Important opportunity

Imagine being able to cut your chance of dying prematurely by 40 percent or more. Put another way, there is a huge opportunity to increase your health span—if not always your life span—by about 40 percent. The key is to take personal responsibility for your health. Too often we like to put too much blame on doctors and the health-care system, and disregard the fact that about 40 percent of our health depends squarely on our lifestyle.

Clearly quitting smoking is one sure way to improve your health span. This is one area where the news is good. Smoking has declined generally in the United States, from 57 percent of adults in 1955 to 23 percent in 2005, although a small uptick to 25 percent occurred between 2006 and 2010.[10] Since a majority of us do not smoke, that brings us to perhaps the single greatest opportunity there is to improve your health—caloric restriction. While there are different forms of fasting, the underlying principle behind scientific fasting is simply profound: eating less could prolong your life and will definitely increase the disease-free period of your life.

In reviewing more than seventy years of research on the role of caloric restriction (CR) on health, I discovered overwhelming evidence that caloric restriction or fasting prolongs the life span of animals, from small creatures all the way up to primates. And while scientists are continuing to investigate the possible role of fasting in human health, most credible research has found significant improvements in health markers in humans and other primates. Later I will go into detail about how scientists conduct these tests and what they are looking for. But suffice it to note at this point that CR research has reached a fairly mature stage. The consensus emerging in the scientific community is significant; namely, that *eating less could save your life or make it much healthier.*

This book is not about prescribing specific diets, although I will offer some general suggestions based on the results of these findings. Nor is this book about weight loss, although eating less will almost surely help you lose weight. It is also not about using fasting to cure existing diseases, although fasting in some cases may help the healing and regeneration process. This book is about fasting intentionally for a healthy and spiritually wholesome life.

Your "response-ability"

The opportunity to positively impact your health also comes with a responsibility to act. In fact, the biggest advantage of CR—unlike exercise—is the opportunity to do little or nothing. Just eat less by skipping a meal or two occasionally. Exercise and dietary considerations are two of the most important behavioral health determinants, yet research has shown that the single most important dietary factor is to skip a meal or two every now and then. In other words, eat less and live better.

You have the ability to fast occasionally. Except for those with health problems, almost everyone can and should fast. Your health depends on it. Even if you are not a religious person, you can fast for the sake of your health. And if you are a person of faith, now is the time to get back to this age-old spiritual discipline. It will help your body and soul heal in ways that will surprise you. I have dedicated a whole chapter to discussing the possibilities that exist when fasting for health purposes is intentionally integrated into moments of spiritual renewal.

In recent years one of the popular books embraced by our culture is *The Seven Habits of Highly Effective People* by the late Stephen Covey. With more than fifteen million copies sold in thirty-eight languages (and another 1.5 million audio copies), it is one of the best-selling nonfiction books in history. Part of the book's popularity derives from the challenge that Covey threw at all of us: there is a space between the stimulus (what happens to us) and response (what we do about it). That space is where we can choose how to respond. In other words, we are capable of changing our path in life. We are capable of choosing what to do about our health. That is one of the unique things that make us human. Don't surrender this ability to choose your response about one of the most important health determinants. Whether you are overweight or not, we all need to stay in good health. There is abundant scientific evidence that eating less or fasting periodically could profoundly impact our health. So what is stopping you from doing something?

There is no such thing as gaining "something for nothing." As with all new habits, fasting may be painful at first. It may not be easy skipping a breakfast when you have gotten used to eating every morning. Fasting a whole day may seem almost impossible—that is, until you actually try it. Skipping sweets and junk foods and living only on vegetables, fruits, and whole grains for a few days or longer may seem daunting. But it can be done. More than seventy years of research from some of the world's most brilliant minds supports its practice. In other words, the facts are on your side.

Don't attempt to start in an overly ambitious manner. Initiate a fasting journey slowly and progressively. I have a few suggestions that may be helpful; however, no matter what someone else says or what examples they offer from their experience, your journey is just that—yours. Embark on it slowly, deliberately, cheerfully, and intentionally. Find out what works for you and adjust accordingly. It is *your* life, *your* journey, and *your* health. I won't be presumptuous enough to assume that I know what is best for you. My only goal is to give you some of the information currently available on fasting's nature, substance, and duration. It is your decision if, when, and how you will embark on this journey. I feel the facts will be persuasive enough to prod you to start, but that is where my role ends. The rest is up to you.

We can only imagine the health revolution that will come to our nation if people take behavioral matters into their own hands and start a fasting lifestyle. Imagine reducing the risk of cancer, stroke, diabetes, cardiovascular diseases, and possibly neurodegenerative diseases by 20 to 50 percent. That is the vision driving the release of this work, which simultaneously presents a huge opportunity and huge responsibility.

It serves no use to read the facts supporting fasting if you don't intend to fast. You cannot be an author until you have written the book. You cannot reap dividends until you have invested. The health benefits are just that: benefits. Fasting is the cause, and health is the effect. Knowing about something isn't the same as experiencing it. Learning and doing are not quite the same. One leads to the other, but you can learn all the facts in the world without doing anything about them. The world is filled with folks who have a lot of knowledge but do not act on it. Those who have made a difference in life are those who have taken a fact—even a simple one—and done something about it.

A precautionary principle

A precautionary principle in good science stresses the "wisdom of acting, even in the absence of complete scientific data, before the adverse effects on human health or the environment become significant or irrevocable."[11] Let us agree that while the studies on humans are not yet conclusive, the overwhelming evidence from animal and primate studies thus far adequately justifies taking the precautionary step of periodic fasting. Then it behooves us to develop a consistent, workable plan.

As another group of scientists summarized the situation after an extensive review of the health benefits of fasting: "Whether current positive results will translate into longevity gains for humans remains an open question. However, the apparent health benefits that have been observed with CR suggest that regardless of longevity gains, the promotion of healthy aging and disease prevention may be attainable."[12]

Given the promise of fasting, particularly during the staggering health crisis that burdens the American system, initiating a plan would seem a wise and prudent course of action. To paraphrase a familiar commercial: "Your stomach deserves a break today."

Chapter 3

SCIENTIFICALLY SPEAKING

Fasting is the greatest remedy—the physician within.

—Philippus Paracelsus, MD (1493–1541)
One of the three fathers of Western medicine[1]

FASTING REFERS TO THE TERM I INTRODUCED IN chapter 2: caloric restriction or intermittent fasting. For those involved in research on successful aging and dietary impact on health, fasting for improved health and longevity means controlled reduction of dietary energy intake of an individual (or animal, in animal model studies) by 20 to 40 percent of customary intake.

I have chosen to call this caloric reduction, or fasting for short. For the purpose of this discussion, and in accurate reflection of the decades of scientific research done in this area, CR means a reduction in energy intake without lowering the nutritional value the body needs.

Scientists generally classify calorie reduction in three broad categories:

1. Caloric restriction, the sustained 20 to 40 percent reduction just mentioned.

2. Alternate-day fasting, also known as intermittent fasting. As the name implies, this is a situation where one eats normally one day, and the next day either reduces intake or eliminates food altogether. This is an alternative to CR, since scientists believe that for many people, continuous sustained CR is stressful and may not prove feasible in the long run. Hence, they expect the process of alternating fasting with normal meals to be more sustainable.

3. Dietary restriction (DR). This is a situation where one or more macronutrient components (such as proteins or carbohydrates) are reduced without significant reduction in total caloric intake. An interesting result has emerged from DR research. While carbohydrate and lipid restriction do not offer any significant health or life span benefits in measurable health biomarkers, protein reduction increases life span in animal studies by as much as 20 percent.[2] Specifically this benefit is believed to be mainly due to reduction in one protein-rich amino acid called methionine. While studies in this area are ongoing, what they should do is serve as a check on the wanton pursuit of every weight-loss craze

that comes along. Long-term health and the delay of age-associated diseases are more important than short-lived weight control. Having the discipline to say no to food intermittently may be a much better approach in the long run.

Reduced energy intake

No matter what category or label scientists give it, the point is clear: reduction in calorie intake can literally save your life. The willingness and ability to adopt a lifestyle change that reduces your overall energy intake while maintaining adequate nutrient intake is key to delaying major diseases and ensuring a healthy, happy life.

For some people, being able to fast two or three times a week may work. I have friends who fast from morning until 6:00 p.m. every Monday, Wednesday, and Friday. You notice that this is similar to what anti-aging scientists call alternate-day fasting. You may begin by fasting only on Fridays. That is a start—an important one that could boost your health.

I started by fasting every Friday and Sunday for several years. Later I fasted every Sunday, plus three other days of complete fasting during that month. Today I basically do more of what researchers call calorie restriction. I have reduced my overall energy intake by about 30 percent. One week of every month I follow a restricted diet where I eat only fruits and vegetables (and sometimes nuts) until 7:00 p.m. and then enjoy a full meal for dinner.

Magic health pill?

Due to the challenge of self-discipline involved in following a calorie-restricted lifestyle, some scientists are also testing certain chemical compounds for their ability to extend life span or induce delays of age-associated diseases. Some of these—specifically a nutrient material called resveratrol and a drug called rapamycin—have been shown to mimic to some extent the health benefits of fasting.[3] As a result, there are efforts now to develop some of these as alternatives to calorie reduction. After all, "Take a pill a day and live longer" appears to be a much more attractive promise than disciplining our behavior and reducing calorie intake.

However, as we have seen with every man-made drug ever invented, no drug can replace the behavioral component of health determination. Choosing a fasted lifestyle that works for you may require diligence, planning, and consistency. Ultimately, though, science has shown that a healthy lifestyle, including a fasted lifestyle, works over the long-term. The powerful benefits of hormesis and reduced oxidative stress that stem from calorie reduction will be difficult to replace with a pill. To be sure, the time may come when we need to take some of these pills to augment the health benefits, but they likely are not sufficient to replace calorie reduction—think obesity and associated diabetes, cancer, and cardiovascular complications. In the long run calorie reduction is the only method that makes sense, medically speaking.

Proof it works

After reviewing several scientific publications—both original research and review articles—I have reached a simple but profound conclusion: there is sufficient scientific evidence to take fasting seriously at a personal level. Given what we know today about the effects of fasting or calorie reduction on health and the aging process, it is surprising that many individuals remain unaware of this simple, free, and natural approach to improving health. Realizing the benefits of calorie restriction isn't magic, but an idea grounded in science. Numerous scientific studies reveal this works on mice, monkeys, and human beings.

While scientists sometimes get lured away by the attractive, esoteric nature of scientific pursuits, it is so easy to forget that real people's lives are at stake. So, let us leave scientists to continue their study and debate about whether CR can extend human life. While we don't know that for certain, most credible studies show that CR improves most important biomarkers of health. They range from reduced adiposity (namely, obesity) to cardiovascular (heart health) biomarkers. In the rest of this chapter I will provide an overview of some of the many studies showing the benefits of calorie reduction on primates and on humans. (In later chapters I will discuss in detail the effects of fasting on reducing your risk for specific diseases, such as diabetes, cardiovascular disease, and Alzheimer's disease.)

These results demand immediate action from everyone. They call us to not only take action, but also to help our loved ones do the same. In developed countries we are literally eating ourselves to an early grave. Most religions teach moderation and call for periods of fasting to train oneself to refrain from self-indulgence and connect with a larger perspective on life. However, my discussion of fasting is aimed at showing its benefits, whether you are a person of faith or no faith. For all the talk about the so-called dichotomy between religion and science, it seems that fasting presents one of those rare opportunities where religion and science seem to agree. Whether motivated by faith or by health, the important thing is that careful scientific studies now show that the age-old practice of fasting regularly does have a profound, long-range positive influence on our health.

As you review the following research summaries, I will hope it will inspire you to draw up a plan of action. Life is too short to eat your way to a premature death. There is more you are called to be and to do. You may not have all the time in the world to visit the gym every day; the kind of job you have may necessitate not being as physically active as you would like. (Still, you should strive to exercise regularly and be as physically active as possible for your circumstances.) However, no matter how intense your desk-bound work schedule or flexibility to work in visits to the gym or health club, you *can eat less*. Fasting intermittently while still getting adequate nourishment is something everyone can do.

Clinical studies on primates

In the July 2009 edition of *Science* a group of bio-medical research scientists from the Wisconsin National Primate Research Center at the University of Wisconsin published the results of a twenty-year study aimed at investigating the effect of calorie reduction on rhesus monkeys.[4] The significance of this report: for the first time it demonstrated the effect of prolonged fasting on primates, the closest species to humans. Even though scientists were convinced from extended research that caloric restriction does increase health span and life span in lower animals, they weren't quite sure if this was the case with primates and humans. They wanted to test this hypothesis with primates.

After two decades of study involving monkeys kept at moderate CR, R. J. Colman and his coworkers learned that animals on CR lived longer than those on a regular diet—80 percent survived with a restricted regimen, compared to only 50 percent of those on a normal diet. Perhaps even more importantly they also discovered CR significantly lowered the incidence of age-associated diseases in those monkeys kept on a regular fasting diet, compared to those fed normally. Specifically the results showed that incidence of diabetes, cardiovascular disease, cancer, and brain atrophy were significantly reduced in animals that fasted. After careful examination of their data, here is one of these scientists' conclusions: "Given the obvious parallels between rhesus monkey and human, the beneficial effects of CR may also occur in humans."[5] This prediction is supported by studies of people on long-term CR, who show fewer signs of cardiovascular aging. Later I will examine in detail the positive effects of fasting on diabetes, cancer, and heart attack incidence.

Human studies

The Okinawan connection

Okinawa is a Japanese island located in the Pacific Ocean roughly four hundred miles south of the rest of Japan. For many years scientists have observed that people living on this small, somewhat isolated island have the longest life expectancy of any group of people—both in Japan and the rest of the world. The Okinawan people also show the lowest risk for major age-associated diseases.[6] For a long time this puzzled scientists, who wanted to know what was responsible for this remarkable phenomenon, especially among older generations.

In 2007 a team of biomedical researchers from the United States and Japan published the first-ever comprehensive, epidemiological studies on the Okinawan phenomenon.[7] Among other things, they set out to confirm whether Okinawans indeed live longer, healthier lives than most other people groups around the world. They also set out to investigate the dietary regimen of older Okinawans to ascertain if caloric restriction played a role in their healthy aging and prolonged life span. Their results, published in the *Annals of the New York Academy of Sciences*, suggest that the answer to both questions is "yes."

For example, they learned that the average diet of senior Okinawans (especially until the 1960s) averaged about 11 percent fewer calories than Japan's national average. They also found out that the average diet of Okinawans consisted of vegetable-laden, low-calorie meals, such as sweet potatoes and green and yellow vegetables. Equally notable:

how their natural diets were rich in vitamins C and E, folate, and vitamin B_6 (as much as 289 percent, 190 percent, 295 percent, and 221 percent higher, respectively, than the daily recommended intake). In simple terms the Okinawan people live longer and healthier lives because—among other factors—they practice calorie restriction as part of normal life.

Human experiment

Dr. Roy Walford and a team of scientists from the Department of Pathology and Department of Surgery and Neurology at the University of California at Los Angeles (UCLA) School of Medicine published a number of reports on a two-year-experiment. As part of other goals of the Biosphere 2 project, they conducted tests on human beings to test the effects of calorie restriction on humans—perhaps the longest-running of such tests on people.[8] The results were published in a number of reputable journals.

Four men and four women ranging in age from twenty-seven to sixty-seven lived in a closed ecological space called Biosphere 2, located near Tucson, Arizona. These eight people agreed to live together and grow virtually all their food inside this biospace for two years. Water and nearly all air and organic matter were recycled inside this living space for that span of time. Because they were constrained to this space and had to grow their own food, there was only so much available. Consequently, by default, they had to adapt to a restricted caloric intake for those two years. However, although their diet consisted of fewer calories, it was still rich in nutrients. At the end of the experiment the men showed an average weight loss of 18 percent, while the women sustained an average 10 percent decrease in weight.

In terms of health, these scientists observed the same kind of health benefits that CR has always conferred on rodents and other animals—improved health, slowed aging process, and lower incidence of disease. The scientists took blood samples from these humans before, during, and after those two years. Then they analyzed them for health biomarkers that are standard in the biomedical field, such as glucose, blood lipid, glycosylated hemoglobin, and insulin. The summary of these tests showed that fasting has the same beneficial effect on humans as observed previously on other vertebrates.

Controlled clinical study

It is possible to dismiss the Okinawa epidemiological study as merely observational. Certainly, while such studies provide a valuable insight to the role of caloric restriction in healthy aging, it is no doubt limited in the conclusions we can draw from that. This is why a group of medical researchers from reputable medical research centers across the country have since embarked on the first-ever comprehensive, randomized clinical trial to test the effects of caloric restriction on human health—and possibly on longevity.

The Comprehensive Assessment of the Long-Term Effects of Reducing Intake of Energy (CALERIE) is sponsored by the National Institutes of Health (NIH). This is currently the largest and most trusted study on the role of calorie restriction on human health. When the NIH commissioned this study, one of its major goals was to investigate whether fasting can actually prolong human life. Since almost all other studies on lower animals had shown that fasting tended to prolong life span, they wanted to determine if this could be true for humans.

Phase 1 of this study has concluded. This phase of the study showed that fasting does improve important bio-markers of health, some of which will be discussed shortly. In fact, spurred by promising results from phase 1 trials, this study has now progressed to phase 2.[9] The second phase, currently in data collection and analysis stage, is aimed at validating and confirming earlier results, by extending fasting period and adopting uniform testing parameters across all clinical sites. While the question of whether fasting extends life span for humans remains rather inconclusive, these NIH-sponsored studies indicate that fasting does improve health span. These studies show that fasting reduces the risk for various life-threatening diseases, as well as improving biomarkers of health. Many of the scientists involved in the first phase of this study have published their results. Below is a brief summary of some of their findings as published in peer-reviewed journals, along with the results of other related studies. I am using the article headlines to provide you with a quick picture of their conclusions, even if you don't read the full summary (feel free to check these articles for yourself).

- "Caloric restriction improves memory in elderly humans."

Scientists from Germany set out to test if caloric restriction, which has improved cognition in lower animals, could be beneficial for cognitive function in elderly humans. The result of their study was published in the *Proceedings of the National Academy of Science*.[10] Their conclusion? They found a significant increase in verbal memory scores for those with restricted calorie intake (a mean increase of 20 percent, P < 0.001). And this improved verbal memory ability correlated with decreases in fasting plasma levels of insulin and high sensitive C-reactive protein. This was most pronounced in participants who adhered closely to the restricted diet. This study effectively demonstrates the beneficial effects of scientific fasting on memory performance in healthy elderly people.

- "Caloric restriction alone and with exercise improves CVD in healthy non-obese individuals."

This is the headline on the article published by Michael Lefevre and coworkers in 2009 as part of the CALERIE project.[11] I will still discuss this article in more detail due to the significant findings it made regarding the effects of fasting on the heart. The purpose of their study was to determine the effect of fasting (caloric restriction) for six months with or without exercise on cardiovascular disease (CVD) risk factors. Based on that, they made a ten-year estimate of CVD risk in healthy non-obese men and women. After careful analysis of their data, their conclusion was that—considering positive changes in lipid and blood pressure observed in those who fasted—caloric restriction with or without exercise favorably reduces risk for CVD, even in already healthy non-obese individuals, especially if that fasting induces weight loss as well.

- "The effect of caloric restriction and glycemic load on measures of oxidative stress and antioxidants in humans: results from the CALERIE Trial of Human Caloric Restriction."

Many believe that decreasing oxidative stress and increasing antioxidant defense may be one mechanism by which fasting increases health span. So a group of researchers at the Human Nutrition Research Center on Aging at Tufts University in Boston decided to study whether fasting (10 percent or 30 percent CR) helps to increase the human body's antioxidative defense.[12] The results of their six-month study appeared in 2011. Their conclusion was that short-term caloric restriction in moderately overweight people results in some positive biomarkers of antioxidant defense.

- "Effect of 6-month calorie restriction on biomarkers of longevity, metabolic adaptation, and oxidative stress in overweight individuals: a randomized controlled trial."

The goal of this study was to investigate the effect of prolonged calorie restriction on biomarkers of longevity or markers of oxidative stress, or reduction on metabolic rate beyond that expected from reduced metabolic mass in humans (12.5 percent CR with about 12.5 percent increase in exercise also). Their conclusion was that two negative biomarkers of longevity—fasting insulin level and body temperature—were favorably reduced by prolonged caloric restriction, demonstrating the health benefits of fasting.[13]

- "Calorie Restriction Increases Muscle Mitochondrial Biogenesis in Healthy Humans."

Caloric restriction without malnutrition is known to lower free radical production by the mitochondria. In order to determine if CR lowers free radical production by the mitochondria in humans, a group of scientists (as part of the CALERIE team) undertook a clinical randomized trial involving healthy humans. Those who participated in CR, with or without exercise, had increased expression of genes encoding proteins involved in mitochondrial function. This study showed that there is an increase in muscle mitochondrial DNA and a corresponding decrease in both body oxygen consumption and DNA damage.[14]

What this means is that fasting improves mitochondrial function—the energy driving cells—in non-obese people. You may wonder about the relevance of improved mitochondrial function on good health and healthy aging. According to the mitochondrial theory of aging, free electrons are often produced as a by-product of aerobic respiration (within the mitochondria). The problem with these free electrons is that they tend to convert oxygen to highly reactive oxygen species (oxygen radicals). These are capable of reacting with and damaging proteins, lipids, and DNA molecules. If this continues over a long period of time, damage accumulates slowly, leading to early incidence of age-associated diseases, such as cancer and others.

- "Effect of Calorie Restriction With or Without Exercise on Insulin Sensitivity, Beta-Cell Function, Fat Cell Size, and Ectopic Lipid in Overweight Subjects."

The purpose of this study was to determine the effect of fasting on insulin sensitivity, fat cell size, etc., in healthy overweight humans.[15] The scientific community accepts as fact that large adipocytes (fat cells) often lead to insulin resistance, through large deposits of fats in abdominal cavity and around the liver. What these scientists found was that fasting alone or with exercise reverses this trend. What does this mean to the layperson? Simply that fasting dissolves fat and improves your sensitivity to insulin, thereby reducing your chances of contracting type 2 diabetes and other medical conditions.

Chapter 4

WHY FASTING WORKS

To lengthen thy life, lessen thy meals.

—BENJAMIN FRANKLIN[1]

B EFORE I REVIEW INFORMATION ABOUT THE SPECIFIC markers of health that fasting has been shown to improve, let us pause to answer a question that may have arisen as you have read: Why does fasting have such a profound effect on human health? Scientists are still grappling with all the details of fasting to explain this. Many have offered propositions (what scientists like to call "a hypothesis") regarding the impact of fasting on overall health. However, reviewing the available data, it appears for now that the scientific community agrees on two possible explanations:

1. The hormetic effect

2. The fact that fasting reduces oxidative damage.

The effect of hormesis

In one study published in 2008, the researcher wrote about how hormesis in aging refers to beneficial effects resulting from the cellular responses to mild, repeated stress.[2] As an aging (and of course, disease) retardant, hormesis is based on the principle that repeated exposure to mild stress stimulates maintenance and repair processes.[3]

There is considerable evidence from highly controlled studies of laboratory animals that reduced dietary energy intake (either controlled caloric restriction or intermittent fasting) can increase the resistance of the animals' cells to various types of stress.[4]

Mild stress, by the way, appears to benefit the body. For example, have you ever stopped to wonder why exercise is beneficial? Strictly speaking—at least at the biochemical level—physical activity shouldn't be good. Why? It is a well-documented scientific fact that exercise increases the production of various potentially harmful substances in your body.[5] Such substances include reactive free radicals (such as reactive oxygen species and nitrogen species), aldehydes, and acids. During exercise your metabolic rate highly increases, due to up to a twentyfold increase in mitochondrial respiration and oxidative phosphorylation (the process by which the body utilizes oxygen we breath in to break down food into energy molecules that power our being). The combined effect is that prolonged exercise results in formation and accumulation of rather harmful substances in your body.[6] Yet when done moderately and intermittently, exercise produces long-term beneficial effects. What shouldn't be a positive ends up producing a beneficial effect on the whole organism. This paradox provides a good model to explain the positive effect of fasting through hormesis.

Like exercise, fasting is what biologists call a mild stress-producing signal or stressor. According to researcher S. I. Rattan, stress may be "defined as a signal generated by any physical, chemical or biological factor (stressor), which in a living system initiates a series of events in order to counteract, adapt, and survive."[7] This general ability of a living organism to adapt to the repeated presence of a low-intensity stressor by stimulating beneficial (but counter-stressor) effects is generally known as hormesis. In healthy aging research, hormesis refers to beneficial effects resulting from cellular responses to mild, repeated stress—such as fasting.

In other words, the cascading effects you experience after fasting are hormetic, much like the benefits of exercise. Restricting the body's caloric intake, if done mildly and *repeatedly*, serves as a mild "stress" to the body. In return, your body initiates a range of cellular activities to adapt to this stress. Because your body is attempting to release effects to counter this stress signal (normally a bad thing), your body ends up releasing a range of positive cellular and physiological responses. Together, they are more beneficial to the body than otherwise possible.[8]

If you think about it, this makes a lot of sense. Vaccines work in a similar fashion. A doctor injects you with a foreign body, such as a chemical or genetic material (known as an antigen). Because of prior studies, scientists know the antigen will cause the body's immune system to produce certain proteins known as antibodies, which will help fight that invading enemy. Although there are substantive differences between the mechanisms of fasting and vaccination, it is still clear that the overall effect in both cases is beneficial. Is there any scientific proof to back up the claim that fasting has this kind of effect? Yes. Several studies on mice and other animals have shown that fasting helps them to survive heat stress more than those on regular meals, protecting them from damage done by toxic chemical agents.[9]

Scientists involved in research on healthy aging are continuing to investigate the exact mechanism by which fasting works via hormesis. Still, scientific results seem to strongly confirm the following suggestion: animals on caloric restriction consistently show elevated levels of stress-regulating hormones—glucocorticoids and particularly plasma-free corticosterone.[10] Why is this important? Because mammals need glucocorticoids in order to cope with harmful environments.[11] To prove that increased levels of these stress-fighting hormones are not the result of some accident, scientists have observed that fasting helps to prevent cancer in rodents. But when they surgically remove the organ that produces these stress hormones, these rodents lose the ability to prevent cancer through fasting.[12] What this shows is that fasting does something to stimulate adrenaline to produce these stress-regulating hormones. There hormones then work synergistically with other physiological processes to (for example) prevent cancer.

Preventing oxidative damage

A pair of studies illustrate how fasting is further beneficial in reducing oxidative stress, which refers to the imbalance between the production of free radicals and the body's ability to neutralize them through antioxidants. To quote the authors:

- "Caloric restriction decreases the steady-state concentration of the production of oxidative damage to proteins, DNA, and lipids."[13]

- "Recent evidence suggests that antioxidant supplements (although highly recommended by the pharmaceutical industry and taken by many individuals) do not offer sufficient protection against oxidative stress, oxidative damage or increase the lifespan. The key to the future success of decreasing oxidative-stress-induced damage should thus be the suppression of oxidative damage without disrupting the well-integrated antioxidant defense network."[14]

We know that high levels of reactive oxygen species—the aforementioned free radicals—in relation to antioxidant defenses play an important role in causing disease and enhancing the aging process. We also know that perhaps the best way to get all the antioxidant defenses we need is eating more vegetables and fruits. Several studies show there are numerous ingredients in fruits that not only help the body maintain the right balance between oxidants and antioxidants, but also help the body to self-renew and therefore remain healthy. In general people who eat fruits and vegetables, which are rich sources of antioxidants, tend to have a lower risk of heart disease and some neurological diseases. There is also evidence from epidemiological studies that some types of vegetables and fruits in general protect against a number of cancers.

Despite this well-documented knowledge, many Americans neglect fruits and vegetables. One published source noted that "80 percent of American children and adolescents and 68 percent of adults do not eat five portions [of fruits and vegetables] a day."[15] This study also noted the inadequate dietary intake of vitamins and minerals on one hand, and a corresponding, excessive consumption of energy-rich, micronutrient-poor, and refined foods.

Instead, too many people try to find simple alternatives—namely, synthetic antioxidants, such as vitamins C or E supplements. As a result, in an awareness and desire to decrease oxidative stress, slow the aging process, and improve our health, we consume more and more antioxidants—usually the synthetic kind. One researcher notes that supplements represent an annual market of more than $7 billion in the United States alone, and more than $30 billion worldwide.[16] But the more antioxidant supplements we consume, the more it becomes apparent that nothing can take the place of fruits and vegetables. Why? Because studies prove that fruits and vegetables contain numerous antioxidants, including a complex mixture of natural substances that—when combined—provide immense benefits to the body. Here is a short list of some of these natural substances:

- *Green tea, resveratrol, polyphenols, and curcumin*: very good inhibitors of cell proliferation.

- *Grapefruits and garlic*: contain powerful inhibitors of P450.

- *Flavonoids and isoflavonoids* (contained in green tea and other natural plants): powerful antagonists of estrogen and inhibitors of metastases (the ability of cancer or other diseases to quickly spread from one organ or part of the body to another), and inhibitors of angiogenesis.[17]

Contributing to health

Together, studies suggest that these ingredients may have important contributory influence to improved cardiovascular health and decreased incidence of cancer. Both have been observed in individuals who consume a higher volume of fruits and vegetables than those who follow a traditional, meat-heavy diet.

Two studies suggest that antioxidant consumption may not be working as well as we would like for a number of reasons.[18] One reason is that the body has its own well-coordinated antioxidant defense system, which allows only a certain amount of antioxidants to reach its cells. Hence, only a limited number of antioxidants consumed actually reach the body. Second, recent studies have shown that the traditional view of oxidative species and aging as being proportionally related is no longer set in stone. Yes, sustained high levels of oxidative species in the body over a long period of time play a role in causing age-associated diseases. Still, there is no conclusive study that has shown that increased antioxidant levels in the body leads to longevity. In fact, some recent studies are showing that the body does need some levels of reactive oxidants to help it maintain homeostasis.

So, if consuming more antioxidants isn't the answer, what is? First, understand that consuming more antioxidants is only aimed at *suppressing* high levels of oxidants in the body. It is not a *preventive* measure. Many people feverishly attempt to assuage an already bad situation; ironically in many cases the body already has a way of dealing with the problem. (For example, most reactive oxygen species are short-lived and are so reactive that they must react with something quickly enough to be converted to something else.) Instead, you should focus efforts on preventive measures that do not allow introduction of extra reactive oxygen species (ROS), which disrupt the body's balance of oxidant/antioxidant levels. The body has its own well-coordinated antioxidant defense system.

To do that, it is necessary to understand how we become exposed to ROS. Reactive oxygen species are generated in two main ways:

1. One is exposure to environmental agents that produce ROS in the body (such as smoking, UV radiation, pollutants in food and environment.)

2. The second source—and the most important one—is from the body itself, from normal mitochondrial respiration.

As noted in a recent review article: "The cells of all present aerobic organisms produce the majority of chemical energy by consuming oxygen in their mitochondria. Mitochondria are thus the main site of intracellular oxygen consumption and the main source of ROS formation. Mitochondrial ROS sources are represented by the electron transport chain and the nitric oxide synthase reaction."[19] To simplify that for the average reader, in the process of breaking down food to generate energy, the body uses oxygen we take in through respiration. In the process of doing this, oxidant species (which we now know as ROS) are generated. It is like a machine that produces good products yet also leaks oil or gas in the process. The more efficient the machine, the fewer leaks—and hence, fewer problems.

For the body, this leakage is in the form of electrons, which then react with oxygen and oxides of nitrogen to produce these toxic ROS materials. As it turns out, the more food the body has to continuously process to produce energy, the more electron leaks that occur; thus, the more reactive oxygen species produced. This means that the best way to prevent formation of ROS is to help the mitochondria (the body's machine that helps us carry out respiration and energy production) to function efficiently.

The role of fasting

More and more studies are showing that calorie reduction helps to reduce the level of oxidative damage in the body.[20] But it is also somewhat surprising to researchers that this increased level of protection from oxidative damage during CR isn't occurring through production of more antioxidants. Instead it is now becoming increasingly clear that CR provides antioxidant protection through increased efficiency in the function of mitochondria. What this means is that when you restrict energy intake, the body generally welcomes that opportunity to help mitochondrial cells become more efficient. Studies have shown that there is less leakage of electrons in mitochondrial cells during CR. And cells are much better protected from oxidative decay. Again, this is a hormetic response to the mild stress being introduced in the system by fasting.[21]

In fact, after reviewing all the current approaches being used in the developed world to attenuate the effect of oxidative stress, one researcher concludes: "To date, only caloric restriction (with adequate vitamin and mineral intake) has obtained scientifically based results for the prolonging of life. It could be concluded that prevention of mitochondrial ROS generation is a more efficient approach to decreasing oxidative stress (e.g., by CR) than quenching any already formed free radicals with antioxidants, since the lifetime of most aggressive free radicals is very short (e.g., .OH) and they react with the first compound encountered (e.g., protein, DNA)."[22]

In other words, fasting works!

Chapter 5

PREVENTING DIABETES

The standard American diet is full of empty carbohydrates, sugars,
fats, excessive proteins, and calories, and it is low in nutrient content. This diet literally causes us to lose nutrients.... Most Americans
are unknowingly sowing seeds for a harvest of obesity, diabetes, and
a host of other diseases by their choices of food and lifestyle habits.

—DON COLBERT, MD,
AUTHOR OF *REVERSING DIABETES*[1]

T HE INFLUENTIAL RADIOLOGICAL SOCIETY OF NORTH
America stunned the world in late 2011 by issuing a
press release on some of the research presented at its
annual meeting. The eye-opener involved a team of medical researchers from the Netherlands who said they effectively cured fifteen patients with type 2 diabetes (the most
common kind) by placing them on a calorie-restricted
diet for four months. The patients ate a diet of five hundred calories per day. Using magnetic resonance imaging
(MRI) technology, the doctors monitored and analyzed
the patients' cardiac function and pericardial fat—the

lump of fatty tissue outside the heart—before and after the trial. They also monitored patients' body mass index (BMI) by checking the extent of their weight loss. The results showed a decrease in BMI from 35.3 to 27.5; anything over 29.9 is considered obese. Patients also showed a loss of fat around the heart and increased heart function. In medical jargon doctors observed that "pericardial fat decreased from 39 milliliters to 31 milliliters. Their E/A ratio, a measure of diastolic heart function, improved from 0.96 to 1.2."[2]

What is particularly astonishing about this study is that none of these patients required insulin injections again, even a year after they had returned to their regular diets and gained weight. Even after a year their heart function still showed improvement. These results are promising and caught the nation's attention—at least in the medical and scientific communities. However, this study is only one of many in recent years showing that calorie reduction can help prevent diabetes. Or in the case of obese patients with type 2 diabetes at least help with management of the disease.

According to the Centers for Disease Control and Prevention, as of 2014 there were approximately 29.1 million diagnosed cases of diabetes in the United States—mostly type 2 diabetes, and most of them associated with obesity.[3] Obesity and such related health issues as diabetes represent huge health problems for the nation. Yet it is amazing that something as simple as refraining from eating too much can help prevent this problem. Periodic fasting may well shield you from type 2 diabetes. Results from several reputable medical labs and publications offer convincing evidence. Considering the epidemic proportion of obesity and health risks accompanying carrying too much weight, it is surprising that not enough medical practitioners are shouting about the benefits of calorie reduction from their medical rooftops. Yet maybe that isn't that surprising, since medical doctors in developed countries are trained to cure diabetes instead of prevent it.

There is encouraging news, though: more doctors are now sharing helpful tips with patients on how to prevent diseases and remain healthy. Still, these doctors are operating more from the goodness of their hearts and an awareness of their obligation to their patients than from medical school training. Plus, preventive measures such as CR are not necessarily a source of income to pharmaceutical companies and their shareholders (which also happens to be us!). As a result, some of these important results haven't received the kind of medical attention and promotion they deserve. I hope to help bridge this gap.

The CALERIE Study

Although many peer-reviewed, reputable studies show that calorie reduction can significantly reduce the risk of diabetes, I will focus on perhaps the most trusted study conducted in the United States—the National Institutes of Health's Institute on Aging. The NIH instituted comprehensive, nationwide research to investigate through clinical trials the effect of CR on health biomarkers in regards to diabetes, cancer, and cardiovascular and neurodegenerative diseases. As I mentioned previously, phase 1 of this study is completed and results have been reviewed, vetted, and published in highly reputable journals. Mentioned in chapter 3, CALERIE stands for Comprehensive Assessment of the Long-Term Effect of Reducing Intake of Energy. In the medical field the industry-accepted gold standard for medical clinical studies is human double-blind, randomized studies. CALERIE is such a study.

So, what did the results from the first clinical study show, especially in regard to diabetes and insulin sensitivity? After placing 150 healthy non-obese individuals (ages twenty-five to forty-five) on calorie restrictions of 25 to 30 percent, studies found that regular fasting insulin concentration was reduced by 29 percent or more.[4] In lay terms the higher the amount of insulin present in your blood when you are not eating, the bigger the risk of diabetes; this probably indicates you are developing insulin insensitivity. The higher your insulin sensitivity, the healthier you are, and the lower your risk of developing type 2 diabetes. So, people on CR have much higher insulin sensitivity, and a greatly reduced risk of developing type 2 diabetes.

In 2012 two researchers conducted a clinical study in Serbia to test the effect of calorie restriction on people with impaired glucose tolerance. People with defective glucose tolerance are often at high risk for type 2 diabetes and high blood pressure. So, to investigate the effects that low-calorie, high-fiber diets have on these patients, they recruited fifty-five obese persons and divided them into two groups. One group of thirty-five patients followed a low-calorie diet (55–65 percent carbohydrates, 15–18 percent protein, and 22–23 percent unsaturated fats, and 20–40 grams of fiber per day) for twelve weeks. The control group of twenty patients ate their normal diets.

At the end of three months researchers checked subjects' blood pressure, fasting plasma glucose, waist circumference, index homeostatic model assessment (HOMA-IR, a biological method to measure insulin resistance), HDL cholesterol, and triglycerides. The group placed on calorie restriction with a high-fiber diet showed significant reductions in diastolic and systolic blood pressure, fasting glucose, index HOMA-IR (lower insulin resistance), and triglycerides, compared to the group that ate their normal diet. Interestingly the fasting group also experienced an increase in HDL cholesterol (due to inclusion of unsaturated fats in their diet).[5]

What does this all mean? In the words of the authors: "These results suggest that implementation of low calorie-high fibers diet with balanced nutritive elements have a positive effect on visceral obesity, fasting glucose, lipid profile, and hypertension in obese people with impaired glucose tolerance and lead to consecutive lowering of cardiometabolic risk."[6]

This study reflects what researchers from the National Institute on Aging found in a report published in 1999. They summarized results of the effect of calorie restriction studies on monkeys and other primates. The report, titled "Calorie restriction in nonhuman primates: effects on diabetes and cardiovascular disease risk," investigated the role of fasting on diabetes and cardiovascular risks. In all the studies reviewed—including works from their own laboratory—fasting proved effective in reducing blood pressure, body fat, triglycerides, blood glucose, and cholesterol; and increased levels of HDL2B.[7] What is the importance of HDL2B? It is a subfamily of HDLs (high density lipoproteins, or cholesterol). Low levels of this lipoprotein have been correlated with increased cardiovascular disease risk. In regards to diabetes, fasting reduced blood level of glucose, meaning increased insulin sensitivity—a condition that reduces the risk of diabetes.

Obesity problems

Obesity frequently shows up in studies related to diabetes prevention. The reason: it has been established biomedically that huge weight gain increases one's risk of such chronic diseases as diabetes, dementia, heart disease, and certain kinds of cancer—especially breast cancer.[8] So there is little doubt that excessive weight gain is a potential health time bomb. That's the bad news. The good news: several studies also show that just a modest weight loss (at least 5 percent) can have a significant, positive impact on one's health, especially in reducing the risk of diabetes.[9]

Now, as important as weight control is, we all know that—for many people—accomplishing this is much easier said than done. So, that leads us to the next piece of good news: fasting seems to be effective at helping people lose weight and sustain the loss. Calorie restriction seems to be most helpful, but due to compliance challenges, intermittent fasting (fasting two or three days a week) or alternate-day fasting (fast one day, eat full meals the next) appears to be more practical for many people.[10] One recent review article examined intermittent fasting, alternate-day fasting, and long-term calorie restriction. While the study found that all three forms of fasting help reduce glucose levels, insulin insensitivity, and other indicators of diabetic risk, it showed that sustained calorie restriction is the most effective.

In one recent study conducted in Spain, researchers at a teaching hospital wanted to determine the impact of calorie restriction on severely obese patients in terms of their risk of cardiovascular disease. As stated earlier, persons who are overweight are at a higher cardiovascular risk, characterized by endothelial dysfunction. This simply means that inner layers of their blood arteries are not functioning properly (due to a variety of factors). This leads to high health risks, ranging from hypertension to stroke to diabetes.[11] One way biochemists quantify how well inner blood vessel walls function is to measure postischemic hyperemia index (saRHI), an indirect marker of endothelial function. In general a higher saRHI index is a good sign, and a lower saRHI index is bad.

These Spanish scientists decided to test the effect of calorie-restricted fasting on the levels of saRHI of participating patients. They carried out their study on thirty-four severely obese patients who had been admitted to the hospital. For three weeks these patients followed a very low-calorie diet (about 800 kcal/day). The researchers also recruited obese and non-obese patients and placed them on the same diet. At the end of the study what they discovered was particularly noteworthy: the very low calorie diet had beneficial effects on all three groups in terms of increasing their saRHI. However, the increase was more dramatic in severely obese patients than in obese and non-obese patients, showing that weight loss correlated with the increase in saRHI. In simple terms this study shows that calorie restriction induces weight loss, and this weight loss in return leads to significant improvement in small artery reactivity.[12]

Here is another important discovery from this study: the markers for metabolic and inflammatory performance were also improved. There was significant reduction in blood glucose levels, systolic blood pressure, LDL cholesterol, and other factors. The reduction in those markers also correlates directly with reduction in diabetes risk.

My goal is not to overwhelm you with scientific data, but to present convincing evidence that fasting (calorie reduction, intermittent fasting, alternate-day fasting or other scientifically studied methods) offers immense benefits— not only in the prevention of diabetes, but also in significantly improving the health of diabetic patients. Many of the results are connected directly with weight loss, but in other studies—even when fasting is not accompanied by meaningful weight reduction—there was still significant improvement in the diabetic condition of patients.

Extensive diabetes study

Perhaps one of the largest human studies ever undertaken on diabetes is the United Kingdom Prospective Diabetes Study (UKPDS), organized in the late 1970s by Dr. Robert Turner and colleagues in Oxford, England. It involved more than 5,100 subjects at twenty-three centers across the United Kingdom. Physicians followed up participants in the study for an average of ten years and collected twenty million data items. Results appeared in a series of reports in top peer-reviewed journals.

One aspect focused on the impact of reduced energy intake on newly diagnosed diabetic patients. A report published in 1990, known in brief as the "UK Prospective Diabetes Study 7," reviewed the results of this aspect of low-calorie intake and diabetes. It concerned more than three thousand newly diagnosed diabetic patients who were placed on restricted energy intake. Their average body weight was about 130 percent, plus or minus 26 percent of ideal body weight. At the end of the study patients not only lost weight, but also their fasting plasma glucose levels were significantly lower. The researchers wrote, "The study concludes that though weight loss was important, the most important factor in regulating their blood glucose level and improving their condition was reduction in energy intake irrespective of weight loss."[13]

What is it about fasting that improves the condition of diabetic patients even when they do not lose weight from fasting? A group of doctors in Italy decided to investigate further. Ilaria Malandrucco and eleven colleagues from the College of Medicine at the University of Rome Tor Vergata in Rome, Italy, decided to study the early effects of very low calorie diets on insulin sensitivity in morbidly obese patients with type 2 diabetes. The results of their work were published in 2012.

They recruited fourteen type 2 diabetic patients (seven men and seven women) aged 60.3 years, ± 3.02 years, who had had diabetes for an average of four years. Patients were extremely obese, in good metabolic control, and consented to use a CR diet alone or a diet with oral hypoglycemic agents (type 2 diabetes drugs). The doctors placed them on a very low calorie diet (400 kcal/day) for seven days; they also performed laboratory tests before and after the fast. The parameters they measured included plasma total cholesterol, triglycerides, Hb A1c (measures level of blood glucose), and other blood levels. These researchers noticed a marked improvement in the metabolic profiles of these patients: average weight loss of 3.22 percent (42 percent of this was fat loss), and decrease in plasma glucose and triglycerides.[14] In order words, their diabetic condition improved.

However, this improvement wasn't so much due to increased insulin sensitivity (which remained about the same even though blood glucose levels decreased significantly), but the improvement observed was a result of the effect the low calorie diet had on β (beta) cell function.[15] Simply put, fasting helps diabetic patients by improving the function of beta cells—a type of cells located in the pancreas, whose main function is to store and release insulin. When there is an increase in blood glucose, beta cells respond by secreting some of the insulin they have stored into the bloodstream, which leads to reduced blood gluclose levels. At the same time they produce more insulin for storage. This is an important finding in its own right; namely, the knowledge that *fasting may have some direct impact on proper function of beta cells*. That has great implications for blood glucose. No wonder fasting seems to have such seemingly dramatic effects on type 2 diabetes.

Personal implications

These results are so important it is worth pausing for a moment to consider that these findings are not some esoteric scientific jargon that does not concern you. Science, backed up by the nation's top health institute, strongly suggests that sustained occasional fasting or planned reductions in energy intake can help prevent diabetes. In fact, other studies involving already obese diabetic patients, such as the study I cited at the beginning of this chapter, strongly suggest that sustained calorie reduction can cure diabetes.

A caution: if you are already diabetic, it is a must that you talk first with your doctor before embarking on any calorie-reduction program. Still, scientific results involving CR in preventing or managing diabetes are so encouraging that you should definitely discuss the possibility of medically supervised, controlled fasting. If you are overweight but not yet diabetic, you are fortunate in reading this book. You can take action. Eat less, cut down on your daily calorie intake, and practice periodic fasting. Do it for yourself and for your loved ones.

If you are healthy and have a good body mass index, then keep it up. These studies by NIH were also conducted on healthy, non-obese individuals like you. This means that to avoid excess weight and diabetes in the future, you need to commit to cut down on calorie intake on a daily basis. This is more than a weight issue; it has everything to do with your long-term health. Adopt the method that works for you. It isn't about a weight-loss program as much as it is about reducing your overall energy intake—while still eating a healthy, balanced diet.

Chapter 6

REDUCING CANCER RISKS

Calorie restriction (CR) without malnutrition is the most potent and reproducible physiological intervention for increasing lifespan and protecting against cancer in mammals.

—RESEARCHERS VALTER D. LONGO AND LUIGI FONTANA[1]

CANCER REFERS TO A DISEASED STATE IN WHICH certain abnormal cells in the body start to grow and multiply in an out-of-control manner. While there are close to one hundred different kinds of cancers, they all replicate themselves in a similar fashion. Cells that grow and invade other healthy, normal cells are considered cancerous. When their progress continues unimpeded, the result is serious illness or death.

According to the National Cancer Institute (a branch of the National Institutes of Health), more than 1.6 million new cases of cancer were expected to be diagnosed during 2015 in the United States, with nearly 600,000 people dying from the disease. The most common types were projected to be cancers of the breast, lung and bronchus, prostate, colon and rectum, bladder, melanoma (skin), and half a dozen more.[2] These are sobering statistics—even frightening. Cancer is so prevalent in developed economies that in the United States alone, about 45 percent of men and 37 percent of women are expected to develop cancer in their lifetime. The situation would be hopeless, if recent studies had not provided a genuine ray of hope.

After reviewing current research on the role of fasting and other nutritional interventions in cancer prevention, here is how a pair of researchers summarized their findings: "An important discovery of recent years has been that lifestyle and environmental factors affect cancer initiation, promotion and progression, suggesting that many malignancies are preventable. Epidemiological studies strongly suggest that excessive adiposity, decreased physical activity, and unhealthy diets are key players in the pathogenesis and prognosis of many common cancers. In addition, calorie restriction (CR), without malnutrition, has been shown to be broadly effective in cancer-prevention in laboratory strains of rodents. Adult-onset moderate CR also reduces cancer incidence by 50 percent in monkeys."[3]

Perhaps one of the greatest discoveries of the modern era is the fact that we can literally prevent, or at least reduce the risks of, cancer and other terrible diseases. This occurs through two primary methods: change in lifestyle and reduced exposure to environmentally hazardous agents. Biomedical studies have repeatedly shown that eating a healthy diet rich in fruits and vegetables, engaging in physical activity, and maintaining a healthy weight can significantly reduce the risk of cancer, diabetes, and cardiovascular diseases.

The lifestyle changes of healthy diet, exercise, and healthy weight are interrelated. Still, getting adequate exercise and eating healthy are a problem for most people, even the well-intentioned and highly educated. In developed countries, people tend to consume excesses of energy-dense foods and get less physical activity. This is a deadly combination that fuels the risk of contracting cancer and other deadly diseases. The obesity epidemic is the topic of another chapter, but here I would observe that the seeming helplessness of Western culture to curb excessive eating is continuing to increase the incidence of such life-threatening diseases as cancer.

Fortunately there is one more option that studies have shown can significantly reduce the risk of cancer: reducing calorie intake. Although physical activity is a wise step toward improving health, CR doesn't require exercise. Nor does it require a strict weight-loss program—at least as we traditionally think of such Spartan regimens. Healthy eating is still a must, though, and one way to eat healthier is to incorporate intermittent calorie reductions in your diet. The results from studies on the ability of CR to prevent cancer are so startling that they can only be termed "amazing."

Historic findings

Scientists first documented that fasting may be beneficial in cancer reduction more than a century ago. In 1909 a Japanese scientist published the first scientific paper showing that calorie reduction in mice helped to inhibit the growth of tumors.[4] Since then several other studies have confirmed this early twentieth century observation: calorie reduction inhibits tumor growth in all kinds of animals.

For example, in 1987 a scientist at the National Institutes of Health conducted a thorough review of all relevant studies on the relationship between caloric intake, body weight, and cancer incidence. He chose a total of eighty-two published experiments on fasting and different kinds of cancer. On average, experimental animals had their total energy intake restricted as follows: 29 percent fewer calories, 50 percent less total fat, and 11 percent less protein than animals fed a full, normal diet. At the end of the experiments, the incidence of cancer in animals placed on limited intake was 42 percent lower than in animals fed normally.[5] In fact, when all those studies were combined and averaged, they showed the incidence of tumor occurrence increased with increasing caloric intake and body weight. Those studies showed calorie reductions as modest as 7 to 20 percent had significant cancer-reducing effects as well.[6]

For a while scientists wondered if the interesting results observed in rodents and other animals could be replicated in nonhuman primates such as monkeys and chimpanzees. Thus, in 1989, researchers embarked on a twenty-year-long project to study the effects of calorie reduction in prevention of age-related diseases, such as cancer and cardiovascular diseases, in rhesus monkeys. As noted earlier, their results were published in 2009 in the prestigious journal *Science*, and showed—among other things—that a 30 percent reduction in rhesus monkeys' calorie intake reduced incidence of cancer by as much as 50 percent.[7] These results from a reputable randomized, controlled, peer-reviewed study stunned the scientific community (albeit in a good way).

Indeed, results from this study, along with others like it, were so encouraging that scientists from the National Institutes of Health—in collaboration with other medical research groups nationwide—began to seriously consider the possible effects of CR on prevention of human cancer and other age-related diseases. So, the NIH's National Institute on Aging instituted the first ever randomized clinical trial to test the effect of CR in humans (this CALERIE study was first noted in chapter 3). Usually CR studies involving humans are filled with certain inherent limitations. For example, you cannot just inject humans with cancer to test how they are faring with CR. In addition, ethical requirements mean that you can only restrict the calories of sick patients to certain levels; it may also prove difficult for a sick person to sustain CR for a long time.

With these limitations in mind, phase 1 of this study involved calorie reductions of 20 to 30 percent for six months. At the end of this period researchers checked for biomarkers of health, which predict whether a person can develop cancer, diabetes, or cardiovascular diseases. They found that patients placed on CR had reduced levels of oxyradicals (remember those free oxygen radicals?) and other internal health hazards. High levels of free radicals lead to cancer and other diseases.

Cancer patient studies

These studies could be seen as studies on the potential preventive role of fasting in cancer. But how about cancer patients? Is there any study of humans showing that fasting could be beneficial to them?

In 2009 a group of colleagues from the University of Southern California published a series of case studies conducted on ten cancer patients. The study tested the role of prolonged fasting on recovery of cancer patients undergoing chemotherapy, especially whether fasting had any role in reducing side effects associated with chemotherapy. Note that prolonged fasting means a period of forty-eight to one hundred twenty hours, which is different than short-term fasts of twenty-four hours or calorie restriction.

In this study the three male and seven female patients (ages ranging from forty-four to seventy-eight) voluntarily fasted between forty-eight and one hundred fifty hours before or shortly after chemotherapy. The types of cancer varied, such as breast, ovarian, uterine, and prostate. These scientists noticed a significant reduction in side effects reported, both in frequency and severity.[8]

Anyone who has been through chemotherapy knows that such symptoms as nausea, vomiting, abdominal cramps, mucosis, diarrhea, and weakness are common. Interestingly patients in this study reported fewer side effects than those who did not fast. They also noticed that fasting before or after their chemotherapy did not have any complications or side effects—showing that fasting could be safe even for cancer patients undergoing treatment. Although this is only a set of case studies and needs to be further confirmed through randomized, double-blind clinical trials, the implications of these findings are still worth noting.

What could be the reason for this observation in cancer patients? One plausible explanation is that prolonged fasting results in more profound physiological changes at the cellular level than calorie restriction or short-term fasting. During prolonged fasting, cells essentially switch completely to metabolism based on fats and ketone bodies. This results in reducing pro-growth factors and activation of signaling pathways, which increase cellular resistance to toxins in both human and animal models.

For example, a study done by researcher J. W. Lee and coworkers showed that prolonged fasting in mice protects them against chemotoxicity by reducing the amount of insulin-like growth factor-1 (IGF-1), a growth-factor hormone that has been linked to aging, and tumor risk and progression. Therefore, it seems that fasting protects normal cells by rearranging their energy allocation away from reproduction and growth processes (desperately needed by cancer cells) toward maintenance pathways (needed more by normal cells) whenever nutrients are scarce or lacking.[9] Fortunately the switch to this "protected mode" occurs only in normal cells and not cancer cells, since cancer cells by nature tend to prevent the activation of stress resistance. Hence, during times of induced stress such as prolonged fasting, there is an opportunity to selectively protect normal cells and improve cancer treatment.

A major side effect suffered by cancer patients, especially those undergoing chemotherapy, is myelosuppression.

This is a condition in which bone marrow activity is reduced. When this happens, then there are fewer white blood cells, red blood cells, and platelets. Of course, the result of such decrease is reduced immunity. The reason chemotherapy results in myelosuppression is because it damages the stems cells (regenerative cells) in bone marrow, which then impairs tissue repair and regeneration.

Can prolonged fasting help with this myelosuppression by helping to facilitate regenerative stem cells? Several researchers set out to investigate this question a few years ago, among mice and in human patients. The results of their study were published in 2014. The study showed that fasting increased the body's immunity and regenerative process, with reduced side effects and death associated with chemotherapy. Prolonged fasting reduced circulating IGF-1 levels and protein kinase A (PKA) activity.[10] (PKA refers to a key gene that when it shuts down signals those stem cells to start regenerating.) This study has wide implications for improving immunity and fighting diseases beyond cancer.

In another study involving yeast cells stimulated to express cancer symptoms in mice and engineered to express different kind of cancers, researchers showed that cycles of fasting followed by normal feeding were as effective as cancer drugs in the treatment of the cancer or delaying the worsening of the cancer in yeasts. In animal models used, when periodic prolonged fasting was used in conjunction with cancer drugs, those mice became cancer-free for a prolonged period of time.[11] In the words of the authors, "These studies suggest that multiple cycles of fasting promote differential stress sensitization in a wide range of tumors and could potentially replace or augment the efficacy of certain chemotherapy drugs in the treatment of various cancers."[12]

There are numerous studies in animal models demonstrating the preventive role of fasting against cancer. For example, in 2011 Olga P. Rogozina, coworkers from the University of Minnesota, and a researcher from the Mayo Clinic published the results of their study on the role of fasting in reducing the risk of cancer in mice. They examined the effect of intermittent and chronic (prolonged) calorie restriction on serum adiponectin and leptin levels in relation to mammary tumorigenesis (breast cancer). Several ten-week-old mice were divided into three groups:

- One group ate a normal diet.

- A second group was on a rotation of 50 percent calorie reduction for three weeks (achieved by diet modification—2x protein, fat, vitamins, and minerals), followed by another three weeks of normal feeding, for seventy-nine to eighty-two weeks.

- The third group was placed on repeating cycles of a 50 percent calorie reduction (achieved by reduction in total calorie and energy intake) for six weeks, followed by another six weeks of normal feeding, for seventy-nine to eighty-two weeks.

At the end of seventy-nine to eighty-two weeks, the mice were killed and their blood samples analyzed for mammary tumors. At the end of the study, for animals that were fed normal meals, the incidence of mammary cancer was 71 percent. The calorie-restricted animals showed an incidence of mammary tumors of 35.4 percent, and for those on intermittent fasting, only 9.1 percent.[13] This study provides additional scientific support to the fact that fasting may have some beneficial effects in reducing cancer risks. About 62 percent less risk in a scientific study is hard to ignore, even if it is an animal model.

Calorie restriction is believed to inhibit cancer growth in part by regulating expression of IGF factors, as noted before. So, in 2013 a team of researchers from the University of California at Los Angeles set out to investigate the role of fasting and IGF-1 on prostate cancer. Their study was published in the *International Journal of Molecular Sciences*. Mice models were divided into four groups:

- The first group ate a normal diet.

- A second group was placed on a 40 percent calorie restriction.

- A third group was placed on ganitumab (this drug is a specifically monoclonal antibody that works against IGF-1 factor and is used to treat cancers).

- The fourth group followed a 40 percent calorie restriction in addition to receiving the ganitumab drug.

At the end of the study results showed that the mice on 40 percent calorie reduction had decreased tumor weight, reduced plasma insulin and IGF-1 levels, and increased apoptosis (programmed cell death). On the other hand, even though the cancer drug reduced tumor growth, it had no effect on final tumor weight. The group that had both the drug and calorie restriction showed the best improvement: decreased tumor progression and tumor weight, decreased levels of insulin and IGF-1, and increased apoptosis (programmed cell death).[14] As expected, the control group that followed the traditional diet fared much worse than the groups that received either the drug or calorie-restricted diet.

While NIH and research laboratories continue to investigate the full effect of CR on humans, it is important to note that NIH does not waste its resources on unpromising medical options. There must be something going on for NIH and other agencies to fund these studies, which proceeded to phase 2 trials on humans. If CR can reduce cancer in primates by up to 50 percent, and if NIH thinks this simple lifestyle change has such a potential to prevent a disease as serious as cancer, then it makes sense to look into this at a personal level before it is too late.

Chapter 7

CARE FOR YOUR HEART

In the end it's not the years in your life
that count. It's the life in your years.

—ABRAHAM LINCOLN[1]

NOT ONLY CAN FASTING REDUCE YOUR RISK OF developing diabetes and cancer, but it can also play a role in reducing the incidence of heart attack. In chapter 3, I mentioned the twenty-year longitudinal study at the Wisconsin National Primate Research Center and these scientists' investigation of the effects of CR on rhesus monkeys. One reason they chose rhesus monkeys for this study is because age-associated diseases in rhesus monkeys have been thoroughly studied and documented by this center and other labs nationwide. Secondly, studies show that chronic diseases in rhesus monkey are similar to the ones observed in humans. The most prevalent—diabetes, cancer, and cardiovascular disease—mirror those of people.

Since the age-associated diseases are similar in both humans and rhesus monkeys, the hope is that studying the long-term effects of fasting on monkeys could provide a useful insight on how protracted, controlled fasting might impact humans. As I mentioned earlier, not only did more of the animals on controlled fasting survive much longer (80 percent, compared to 50 percent of those fed normally), the scientists noticed that fasting delayed the onset of age-related diseases in animals.[2]

In a parallel study at the National Institute on Aging (an arm of the National Institutes of Health), researchers investigated the impact of caloric restriction (controlled fasting) on both life span and health span. In 2012 this group published an update in the journal *Nature* to highlight its findings. After many years of research and observation this group concluded that fasting offers extensive health benefits, and called for separation between the health benefits of fasting and its possible life-prolonging effects. In all these studies, not only was fasting beneficial in reducing risk of cancer and diabetes, but it was also especially helpful in reducing incidence of cardiovascular diseases.[3]

It is important to note that the National Institute on Aging study did not offer any conclusive evidence that calorie reduction provided clear life-extension effects. Yet the study found that fasting provided immense health benefits, including cardiovascular health. This is consistent with the findings at the Wisconsin National Primate Research Center. Based on these parallel, twenty-year longitudinal studies, there may be some question about the ability of fasting to extend human or primate life span. Still, there is no doubt that fasting provides sound health benefits that improve health span.

As part of the previously mentioned CALERIE (Comprehensive Assessment of the Long-Term Effects of Reducing Intake of Energy), researchers examined the potential health benefits of fasting in sedentary, non-obese, healthy individuals. But a part of their study focused specifically on the effect of prolonged, controlled fasting on cardiovascular health. The study examined thirty-six humans, each randomly assigned to one of three groups. The control group ate normal meals for six months, the second group did a controlled fast (25 percent reduction of normal energy intake for six months), and a third group reduced its energy intake by 12.5 percent, with a 12.5 percent energy expenditure through aerobic exercises.

Researchers examined cardiovascular risk factors for these groups at three- and six-month timelines, using these figures to estimate ten-year cardiovascular disease (CVD) risk in healthy, non-obese men and women. The results of their study were published in 2009 with a rather telling title: "Caloric restriction alone and with exercise improves CVD risk in healthy non-obese individuals." This conclusion was based on favorable changes in lipid and blood pressure levels, which reduced the risk of CVD.[4] Results from the second phase of these trials were expected to provide more conclusive data regarding the role of fasting in improving cardiovascular health. Meanwhile data from most animal studies show conclusively that calorie restriction does have beneficial effects on heart health.

Risk factors

To better understand the role of fasting in reducing the risk of cardiovascular diseases, let us examine the risk factors and causes of CVD. Atherosclerosis is a major disease condition in which plaque builds up in arteries. Over time plaques—made up of calcium, fats, cholesterol, and other substances—harden and begin to narrow the arteries. The arteries are blood vessels that carry blood (including oxygen and nutrients) to various parts of the body, including the heart, brain, kidney, and other organs. When plaques build up, they narrow arteries and significantly reduce blood flow. The tendency to form blood clots, which further impedes blood flow, is higher. Since atherosclerosis can affect any artery in the body, different diseases may develop, depending on which artery is affected.[5]

Plaque buildup in atherosclerosis is the main cause of three deadly diseases generally grouped as cardiovascular diseases—coronary artery disease, cerebrovascular disease, and peripheral artery disease. Coronary artery disease has to do with sudden rupture of plaques in heart arteries. Plaques in arteries that carry oxygen-rich blood to the heart can rupture and form clots, which may cause the muscles of the heart to die. When this happens, it is known as a heart attack.[6] On the other hand, cerebrovascular disease is caused by rupturing of plaques in arteries that carry oxygen-rich and nutrient-rich blood to the brain. This is what causes a stroke. Finally, peripheral artery disease occurs when arteries carrying blood to the legs become blocked by plaques, which reduces free circulation of blood. This may result in the inability of wounds to heal well, or pain when walking. If this persists, it may lead to amputations.

The following data published by the American Heart Association, and reproduced verbatim, illustrates the seriousness of cardiovascular diseases:

Disease risks

- Cardiovascular disease is the leading global cause of death, accounting for 17.3 million deaths per year, a number that is expected to grow to more than 23.6 million by 2030.

- In 2008, cardiovascular deaths represented 30 percent of all global deaths, with 80 percent of those deaths taking place in low- and middle-income countries.

- Nearly 787,000 people in the US died from heart disease, stroke and other cardiovascular diseases in 2011. That is about one of every three deaths in America.

- About 2,150 Americans die each day from these diseases, one every forty seconds. Cardiovascular diseases claim more lives than all forms of cancer combined.

- About 85.6 million Americans are living with some form of cardiovascular disease or the after-effects of stroke.

- Direct and indirect costs of cardiovascular diseases and stroke total more than $320.1

billion. That includes health expenditures and lost productivity.

- Nearly half of all African American adults have some form of cardiovascular disease—48 percent of women and 46 percent of men.

- Heart disease is the leading cause of death in the world and the United States, killing over 375,000 Americans a year. It accounts for one of every seven deaths in the nation.

- Someone in the US dies from heart disease about once every ninety seconds.

More on heart disease

- From 2001 to 2011, the death rate from heart disease fell about 39 percent—but the burden and risk factors remain alarmingly high.

- Heart disease strikes someone in the US about once every forty-three seconds.

- Heart disease is the No. 1 cause of death in the United States, killing over 375,000 people a year.

- Heart disease is the No. 1 killer of women, taking more lives than all forms of cancer combined.

- Over 39,000 African Americans died from heart disease in 2011.[7]

Fasting's benefits

So what causes these dangerous plaques to build up in the first place? The major risk factors for atherosclerotic diseases include high low density lipoprotein (LDL) cholesterol, low high density lipoprotein (HDL) cholesterol and high triglycerides levels, high blood pressure, diabetes mellitus, and smoking. Atherosclerosis is believed to start with damage to the endothelium (innermost layer) of arteries, which in turn is caused by high cholesterol, smoking, or high blood pressure.[8] Once the endothelium is damaged, cholesterol is able to enter the wall of the artery, causing white blood cells to be released in order to digest the LDL. Over time progressive accumulation of LDL combines with cells and calcium to form a plaque in the wall of the artery.

Here is where fasting becomes so significant: to date, in almost all studies involving rodents, all these risk factors for CVD (except smoking) were significantly reduced through calorie restriction directly, or through weight loss resulting from fasting. In other words, studies involving rodents conducted for decades show that fasting (calorie reduction or intermittent fasting) consistently reduces bad cholesterol levels, triglycerides, and high blood pressure.

It is true that using rodents for CVD model has its limitations in humans, since CVD type that occurs in humans is different in some ways from CVD models in rats.[9] Still, studies show that similar risk factors predictive of cardiovascular risk—such as oxidative stress—show the same downward spiral during fasting in both animal and human studies. Also important is the fact that similar improvements in CVD have been observed in nonhuman primates, as the two results cited previously show. And in case there is any doubt that these benefits observed in animal models are transferrable to humans, the first phase of the CALERIE study showed that even six-month calorie restriction reduces CVD risks in humans.

There are several more published studies demonstrating the beneficial effects of fasting, or intermittent fasting, on reducing the risk of heart attack. My goal is not to provide an exhaustive review of all reputable articles, but to lay a firm foundation for you to appreciate the immense scientific evidence supporting the idea of the benefits of fasting on cardiovascular health—benefits that apply whether discussing simple animals, nonhuman primates, or humans.

Given this reality, it is time to protect your heart. Studies show that people who fast periodically or generally reduce their energy intake on a daily basis (what some call a "fasted lifestyle") are less likely to experience heart attack. This calls for action. All these studies and health benefits will not mean much unless you start doing something about it. It is time to consider your own unique fasting program, one that will fit your needs and situation. As I have already mentioned, you can simply start by skipping a meal or two regularly. Or you can start by generally reducing your regular food intake by 15 to 40 percent. Or start by fasting once or twice a week during the day before eating a normal evening meal. It doesn't matter how you start. The important thing is to start—today.

Resist the temptation to turn this into another weight-loss fad. That is why I have devoted so much time to showing you the scientific studies that support fasting. I want to avoid the tendency of the public to boil things down into some supposedly simple, seven-step program or a fancy slogan. Fads will come and go, but a personal decision to cut your energy intake and fast periodically will produce lasting results. This is about a lifestyle change that will bring you immense health benefits over the long term.

Chapter 8

BOOST YOUR BRAIN

I fast for greater physical and mental efficiency.

—PLATO[1]

DOES FASTING IMPROVE BRAIN HEALTH AND function? It turns out that a significant number of research studies indicate that fasting can do just this. There is some evidence that calorie restriction or intermittent fasting offers protection against age-related neuronal loss and neurodegenerative disorders such as dementia, Alzheimer's disease, Huntington's disease, and Parkinson's disease. Caloric restriction and intermittent fasting have also been shown to reduce the risk of stroke and depression. These are significant statements to make about the role of fasting in improving brain health. In a 2014 TED talk Mark Mattson—chief of the Laboratory of Neurosciences at the National Institute on Aging—commented, "We think the reason—the main take-home message of this talk is that fasting is a challenge to your brain and your brain responds to that challenge of not having food by activating adaptive stress response pathways that help your brain cope with stress and risk."[2]

In this chapter I will highlight some of the studies making these correlations between fasting and cognitive function and mood. But first, a brief crash course on the molecular basis for the role of fasting in improving brain health. In other words, in what ways does fasting contribute to health function at the biomolecular level? Although some fairly technical terms are involved, you don't need a degree in biochemistry or pharmacology to understand this. In chapter 4 I reviewed some of the molecular mechanisms involved in health benefits from fasting in general; namely, hormesis (activation of adaptive cellular stress responses), improved mitochondrial function, and antioxidant activity.

While all those mechanisms also apply to neuroprotection, in this chapter I will focus more on other specific cellular and molecular mechanisms of fasting in improving brain health. These mechanisms include increased neurotrophic factor activity and improved neurogenesis, sirtuin activity, neuronal autophagy, protein chaperone activity, ketogenic bodies, and anti-inflammatory effects. But for the purposes of helping readers better understand this section, I will focus on three of those mechanisms: neurotrophic factor activity and neurogenesis, neuronal autophagy, and ketone bodies.[3]

Neurotrophic factors

Neurotrophic factors, sometimes referred to simply as neurotrophins, are growth factors that promote the survival and growth of neurons. This class of proteins promotes growth and development of neurons in the central nervous system and peripheral nervous system. There are about four subclasses of these structurally related factors:

- Nerve growth factor (NGF)
- Brain-derived neurotrophic factor (BDNF)
- Neurotrophin-3 (NT-3)
- Neurotrophin-4 (NT-4)[4]

Their mode of action is to prevent initiation of neuronal-programmed cell death, thereby allowing neurons to survive. Neurotrophic factors also induce and facilitate differentiation of precursor cells to form new neurons. While all these growth factors play important roles, the focus here is the role of brain-derived neurotrophic factor in brain function. Studies indicate now that degenerative diseases of the nervous system may result from insufficient supply of neurotrophic factors, especially BDNF. It is true that a majority of neurons in the human brain are formed prenatally; the hippocampus is one of the few parts of the adult brain that still retain the ability to grow new neurons. This occurs through a process known as neurogenesis. And it is this process that is facilitated by BDNF and other growth factors. BDNF is present in the hippocampus, cortex, cerebellum, and basal forebrain.

A key fact about the hippocampus: it is the region of the brain known to regulate learning, memory, and mood. In addition, the hippocampus is very sensitive and responsive to external stimuli, meaning that the hippocampus can easily activate adaptive response to cellular stress.[5] In part, this ability of the brain to change in response to different stimuli is known as brain plasticity.

Many studies have shown some evidence of decreased expression of BDNF in neurological diseases, some of which I will examine in more detail. While studies in this area are ongoing, suffice it to say that numerous reports demonstrate that reduced BDNF levels correlates with several neurodegenerative disorders. Several studies have shown that fasting leads to increased levels of BDNF, and therefore offers some neuroprotection against neurodegenerative diseases implicated in low levels of BDNF, such as Alzheimer's and Huntington's disease.

Neuronal autophagy

To get a better grasp of "brain power," consider its functions and vast network of neurons. Let's review some essentials about the central nervous system (CNS), the brain and the spinal cord:

- The CNS has about 1,000,000,000,000 neurons and 1,000,000,000,000,000 synapses; 62,000 miles of myelinated axons; and 100,000 miles of dendrites; it also has up to 15,000 connections per cell.

- The average neuron may have about 1,000 synapses.

- The average axon may synapse on about 1,000 neurons.

- Each of the 100 billion neurons may have
  the processing capacity of a medium-sized
  computer, computing about a thousand
  multiplications and additions every ten
  milliseconds.[6]

There are literally billions of neuronal activities going on at any given time. Dendrites serve as a source of informational input to the neuron while synapses serve to relay information between neurons (Figure 1). The axon is responsible for transferring proteins and organelles over significant distances in the nervous system, making the quality control of proteins critical for proper neuronal function. In addition, synapses require high-energy demand and protein turnover for proper functioning. More importantly, neurons are postmitotic and do not replicate, meaning they are predisposed to accumulate toxic proteins and impaired organelles.[7]

While neurogenesis, facilitated by neurotropic factors, involves preventing death of needed neurons, neuronal autophagy means facilitating death of neurons that are no longer needed or that have become loaded with toxic proteins. Due to the importance of tightly controlling proteins and organelles in the neurons, neuronal autophagy seems to be regulated separately from that of non-neuronal cells.[8]

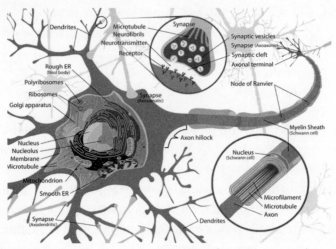

Figure 1: Image of a Neuron[9]

What does this ability of the body to self-destroy damaged neurons that have accumulated toxic proteins or dysfunctional organelles have to do with neurodegenerative diseases—namely, such serious diseases as Alzheimer's disease, Parkinson's, Huntington's, and amyotrophic lateral sclerosis (often called Lou Gehrig's disease)? As it turns out, quite a bit. Intracellular aggregation of proteins and damaged organelles are common features of neurodegenerative diseases.[10] This means that in the course of these diseases, toxic protein aggregates that have accumulated within specific types of neurons lead to their malfunctioning and ultimately neuronal death.

In essence, any process that increases the ability of the body to effectively and selectively destroy those damaged neurons (known as autophagy) improves the prognosis for neurodegenerative diseases or reduces the risk of their early onset. Interestingly one of those experimentally proven interventions that seem to increase neuronal autophagy is fasting. In a study conducted in 2010, researchers showed that fasting in mice "causes a rapid and profound upregulation of autophagy in the brain."[11]

The experiment was conducted on six-to-seven-week-old male GFP-LC3 mice, which ate a food-restricted diet for twenty-four or forty-eight hours. This process is known to induce fatty change and autophagy in the liver. Scientists freely provided water to these experimental mice. Then they euthanized these mice and non-fasting control mice. Sections of their livers and brains were prepared, stained, photographed, and analyzed for autophagosomes. Calorie restriction is a well-known scientific way to induce autophagy and upregulates autophagy in many organs including the liver. For years many scientists believed that perhaps the brain is able to escape this effect—probably because it is a metabolically privileged site. But this study shows that autophagy not only works in the brain, but also that food restriction stimulates and upregulates it within the brain as well.[12]

Ketone bodies

Ketone bodies are a group of three compounds that are produced as by-products from fatty acid catabolism in the liver and kidney. They are used as a source of energy, especially for the brain. Under normal circumstances, the brain derives most of its energy from glucose metabolism. However, during fasting periods, glucose level is depleted, so the brain relies more on availability of ketone bodies for energy supply. The three compounds are β-hydroxybutyrate and acetoacetate, and acetone.[13] Although they are called "bodies," they are actually chemical compounds that are soluble in water. As ketone bodies build up in the blood during or immediately after fasting, they cross the blood-brain barrier through monocarboxylic acid transporters, which are proton-linked transporters. Transported ketone bodies then enter neurons either by diffusion or through monocarboxylic acid transporters.[14] Expectedly fasting increases the permeability of the blood-brain barrier to ketones and improves the expression of monocarboxylic acid transporters.

So, what do ketone bodies from fats have to do with brain health? Quite a bit. The brain functions through the ability of excited neurons to transmit signals and process information. So, while neuron excitation is a good thing, overexcitation is bad for neurons, since it tends to destroy them. This means that the brain has to constantly regulate excitation and balance it with a level of inhibition. Two neurotransmitters play this regulatory role. On one hand is glutamate, which is the excitatory neurotransmitter. On the other is gamma-aminobutyric acid (GABA), which inhibits excitation. Significantly in seizures, stroke, and neurodegenerative diseases *there is more glutamate excitation going on,* which is a problem. It can lead to calcium-dependent neuronal injury and death, through generation of reactive oxygen species and damage to mitochondrial bioenergetic function.[15]

So, here is where ketone bodies come in. As far back as the 1930s, studies showed that directly injecting ketone bodies into rabbits stopped chemically induced seizures through inhibition of glutamate release. For decades the mechanism was unknown. However, recent studies involving hippocampus neurons have shown that ketone bodies directly inhibited glutamate-mediated excitation. On the other hand, ketone bodies have also been shown to increase GABA in synapses of rats and even in certain human brains.[16]

Also, another study showed that a combination of β-hydroxybutyrate and acetoacetate at very low millimolar range decreased the production of reactive oxygen species by complex I of the mitochondrial respiratory chain.[17] It is important to note that ketone bodies prevented neuronal injury and apoptosis caused by hydrogen peroxide or by the glutathione oxidant.[18] All of this means that ketone bodies, available either through fasting or by ingesting a ketogenic diet, have neuroprotective effects.

Empirical evidence

Now that I have established a framework for understanding some of the molecular mechanism of action of fasting in improving brain health, I want to examine studies related to depression, mild memory loss, Alzheimer's disease, and stroke.

Fasting and depression

The federal Centers for Disease Control and Prevention (CDC) estimates that about one in ten Americans suffer from depression at any given time.[19] According to the CDC, depression ranges from mild or moderate depressive disorder ("other depression") to major depression. Referencing a study, its report says: "Participants were considered to have major depression if, for 'more than half the days,' they met at least five of the eight criteria, including at least one of the following: 1) 'little interest or pleasure in doing things' or 2) 'feeling down, depressed, or hopeless.' The [other] criteria were: 3) 'trouble falling asleep or staying asleep or sleeping too much,' 4) 'feeling tired or having little energy,' 5) 'poor appetite or over-eating,' 6) 'feeling bad about yourself or that you were a failure or let yourself or your family down,' 7) 'trouble concentrating on things, such as reading the newspaper or watching television,' and 8) 'moving or speaking so slowly that other people could have noticed... or the opposite: being so fidgety or restless that you were moving around a lot more than usual.' Participants were considered to have 'other depression' if they met two, three, or four of the eight criteria [for major depression listed above], including at least one of the following 1) 'little interest or pleasure in doing things' or 2) 'feeling down, depressed, or hopeless.'"[20]

According to 2009–2010 estimates, about eight million Americans a year are rushed to hospitals or emergency rooms in ambulances with depression as the major diag-nosis, with more than 39,000 suicides resulting from depressive disorders. Antidepression medications rep-resent the third most common prescription taken by Americans of all ages; for the most recently available data for the period 2005–2008, the rate of antidepres-sant use in the United States increased about 400 per-cent.[21] Without a doubt, depression is a major health issue. Additionally the fact that depression is associ-ated with certain chronic diseases such as obesity and stroke makes it an important health risk that the nation must tackle.

So, what does fasting have to do with depression? For many years clinical researchers have found a positive correlation between fasting and mood improvement in patients. The staff at the department of internal and complementary medicine at Immanuel Hospital in Berlin, Germany, has done quite a bit of work in this area. In 2006 they conducted a study (among others) that showed patients put on a fasting regimen experienced improvement in mood.[22] Conducted in a nutritional ward, doctors placed thirty-six patients on an eight-day modified fast (300 kcal/day). They then took daily measurements of ratings of mood, weight, and levels of leptin and cortisol four times within a two-week study period. Fasters showed a more pronounced decrease of leptin (58 percent vs. 20 percent; P < 0.001) and a 17 percent increase in levels of cortisol, the "stress hormone" (P < 0.001). Mood ratings increased significantly toward the later phase of fasting (P < 0.01) but were not related to weight loss, leptin depletion or cortisol increase. The study concluded that fasting induces specific mood enhancement, but indicates that the physiological pathway may not be due to cortisone increase or leptin reduction.[23] In fact, in an earlier study in 2002 involving the effects of fasting (250 kcal/day) for two weeks in fifty-two patients with chronic pain and metabolic syndrome, researchers found that over 80 percent of fasters showed a rapid decrease in depression and anxiety scores, with an average weight loss of 14.6 pounds.[24]

In another human study conducted in Malaysia, thirty-two men with an average age of 58.8 ±5.1 years were placed on a 25 percent calorie restriction in addition to two days per week of religiously based fasting. At the end of the three-month study those men scored lower in tests for depression.[25]

So, how does fasting work to improve mood and reduce depression? Remember BDNF, that brain-derived neurotrophic factor? BDNF has been demonstrated to be an important biomarker for major depression. Several clinical studies have shown that serum levels of BDNF are significantly lower in patients with major depressive disorder. What's more, antidepressant treatments reverse this effect. It has been shown that antidepressants appear to work by increasing the level of BDNF in the hippocampus.[26] In fact, a study by two researchers showed that direct infusion of BDNF into the hippocampus is enough to elicit an antidepressant-like effect in animal models of depression.[27] And to further show that BDNF has a direct role in antidepressant efficacy, mouse models in which the BDNF gene had been mutated or deleted completely did not even respond to antidepressants.

BDNF also produces antidepression effects in the brain and promotes neurogenesis.[28] Today the scientific community seems to have reached a consensus that neurotrophic factors—especially BDNF—play an important role in signaling pathways in the hippocampus and prefrontal cortex involved in ameliorating depression. Equally important is the finding from these studies that stress suppresses BDNF levels in the hippocampus and prefrontal cortex. To simplify: these studies show that almost all antidepressant treatments increase

BDNF synthesis and improve BDNF signaling within the brain's hippocampus and prefrontal cortex. This means that increasing BDNF within the brain correlates with improved mood and, hence, decreased anxiety and depressive disorder.

You may wonder if any evidence indicates that fasting improves levels of BDNF in depression patients; the answer is yes. Studies suggest that the beneficial role of fasting on depression is due to increased BDNF levels observed during fasting. Fasting has been shown to cause an increase in BDNF involved in the regulation of serotonin metabolism, synaptic plasticity, improved cognitive function, and increasing the brain's ability to resist aging.[29] Another mechanism thought to aid mood during fasting is the increased production of ketone bodies, which have been demonstrated to improve mood and decrease pain sensation.[30]

It is also possible that some of the effects of fasting on mood may be explained simply by hormesis. For example, scientists have surmised that prolonged fasting acts as a strong physiological stimulus equivalent to a biological stress, activating the hypothalamic-pituitary-adrenal axis (HPA, the "stress axis"), which produces several adaptive hormones and neurotransmitters.[31] Although the precise biological mechanism of activation may be unclear, it is believed to include reduced availability of cerebral glucose, and reduced insulin and leptin levels.

Taken as a whole, these studies suggest that fasting induces a range of biochemical and physiological processes that elicit a beneficial effect in mood improvement, leading to observed improvement in depressive symptoms.

To be clear: these studies are in their early stages. There are still no credible, randomized, controlled clinical trials to study the effectiveness of fasting on major depressive disorder. Most of the current studies are on animal models. So, until we have more than a few exploratory studies involving human subjects, these studies need to be treated with a dose of skepticism.

Still, every biomedical breakthrough in humans has followed the same sound scientific experimentation and peer-review process starting with various animal models. While I am not suggesting you embark on a protracted fast to cure major depressive disorder without consulting your doctor, initial results are that sustained, preventive fasting does offer benefits, even mood improvement.

Fasting and memory improvement

As far back as 1987 researchers demonstrated that calorie restriction in mice resulted in improved memory and motor coordination. One set of mice ate a normal diet (95 kcal/week), while a second set of mice followed a limited diet (55 kcal/week) for about thirty-five months. The scientists observed that the mice on a restricted diet saw less age-related decline in motor coordination and learning, with their motor coordination enhanced in comparison to the group on a normal diet.[32]

In chapter 3 I mentioned the 2009 study by internal medicine researchers at the University of Münster in Germany, who set out to investigate if such beneficial effects can be observed in humans. To give you a little more detail, they enrolled fifty adults ranging in age from fifty to eighty. In this interventional study they divided the participants into three groups:

- One group (the control) followed a normal diet as before.

- A second group had a 30 percent reduction in calorie intake.

- The third group ate normally, but with a 20 percent increase in unsaturated fatty acids (with no overall increase in fat intake).

The doctors wanted to see if calorie reduction and/or increase in unsaturated fatty acids could lead to improvement in memory. The fasting group showed a 20 percent increase in memory scores/ability (P < 0.001) than the group that didn't reduce calorie intake. They also noticed that this increase in memory ability correlated to increased insulin sensitivity and reduced inflammatory activity.[33]

Increased oxidative stress and impaired energy metabolism, among other factors already discussed, are believed to contribute significantly to neuronal dysfunction and death resulting in memory loss and other neurodegenerative diseases. This interventional study provided some evidence that caloric restriction does have beneficial effects on memory performance in healthy elderly people. This occurs, in part, by improving glucose metabolism, resulting in higher insulin sensitivity and inducement of a range of other cellular adaptive processes.[34]

Alzheimer's disease

Alzheimer's disease has been identified as the most common form of dementia. Dementia is a general term used to describe the loss of memory and other intellectual abilities serious enough to interfere with daily life. Alzheimer's disease is believed to account for between 60 and 80 percent of all dementia cases. According to the Alzheimer's Association about 5.3 million Americans had Alzheimer's disease in 2015; approximately 200,000 individuals were younger than age sixty-five. Women, pay attention: females are particularly at risk. Almost two-thirds of Americans living with Alzheimer's are women. The number is estimated at 3.2 million, compared to 1.8 million men. In fact, the average woman has a greater chance of developing Alzheimer's (one in six) than breast cancer (one in eleven).[35]

It is not clear why women seem to be at greater risk, but that is reality. Alzheimer's is the sixth leading cause of death in the nation, with researchers estimating this disease claims up to 500,000 lives annually. In other words, many of those people wouldn't have died if they did not have Alzheimer's. Between 2000 and 2010 mortality rate for other diseases decreased, but mortality from Alzheimer's increased by 68 percent within the same span of time. In addition, Alzheimer's is the most expensive medical condition to treat. Unless a major medical breakthrough occurs as baby boomers age, the number of Americans aged sixty-five and above with Alzheimer's is projected to skyrocket to about sixteen million by 2050.[36]

Unlike what most people are made to believe, Alzheimer's is not necessarily a disease caused by old age, as though it were a "normal" part of aging. Still, the best known risk is aging. The brain of someone with Alzheimer's is often associated with certain biochemical and physiological changes; mainly, a buildup of extracellular β-amyloid protein, which results in plaque buildup. In addition, there is an aggregation of hyperphosphorylated forms of special structural protein, called tau protein. This leads to biological tangles, called neurofibrillary tangles, and shrinking of the brain.[37]

The Alzheimer's Association's website has a user-friendly, interactive tool about the brain that you may find useful. Think plaques and a twisted mass of tangles in the brain, which can't be good for such sensitive tissue. Synapses, those points where "messages" are relayed from one neuron to another in order to communicate with the body, get affected the most by this buildup of plaques and tangles. They become easily impaired and are ultimately damaged, leading to a range of neurodegenerative conditions.[38] While there is no known cure for this disease, it can be managed medically. That leaves scientists to examine behavioral factors, such as diet and health practices, that could help delay or reduce the risk of Alzheimer's onset. It is in this light that several studies have been conducted to investigate the role—if any—that fasting (calorie restriction or intermittent fasting) may have on reducing the risk of Alzheimer's or even delaying its onset significantly.

Is there any evidence that fasting can reduce the risk of Alzheimer's disease, either from animal or human studies?

Fortunately yes. In 2007 researchers using a transgenic mouse model of Alzheimer's disease demonstrated that a 30 percent calorie restriction resulted in production of more genes associated with neurogenesis, prevented the hippocampus from atrophy, and reduced the production of genes known to stimulate inflammation.[39] In another animal study in 2007 involving mice genetically engineered to have Alzheimer's disease, researchers showed that a 40 percent calorie restriction or intermittent fasting for fourteen months significantly reduced or delayed cognitive decline.[40] Interestingly the improvement in cognitive function is also correlated with significantly reduced levels of β-amyloid protein and phospho-tau (remember those two implicated in causing brain plaque and tangles?).

While there is evidence of improvement in animal models, how about human studies? Clinical studies involving humans are scarce and only beginning to emerge. Still, there are epidemiological studies, which refers to the presence of diseases in large population. One such study in Sweden, completed in 2005, investigated the relation between midlife body mass index and the risk of vascular risk factors, and subsequent dementia and Alzheimer's. Researchers studied more than 1,400 people and followed up on them for twenty-one years.[41] At the end of the study they concluded that being obese at midlife (a BMI greater than 30kg/m2) was directly associated with higher risk of dementia and Alzheimer's disease in particular, even after adjusting for sociodemographic variables, midlife blood pressure, smoking, cholesterol level, and other factors.[42]

In another study conducted in New York, researchers learned that low dietary energy intake was directly associated with decreased incidence of Alzheimer's disease and Parkinson's disease.[43] As you can imagine, these human studies are not yet sufficient to draw any far-reaching conclusions as it specifically relates to ameliorating Alzheimer's in humans. However, studies from animal models and other brain health studies show clearly that fasting does have a beneficial effect on memory and results in reduced levels of plaques and tangles associated with Alzheimer's disease.

Fasting and stroke

After Alzheimer's, the next most common form of dementia is vascular dementia, which occurs after a stroke. So, it is worth discussing stroke in general, and the possible role of fasting in reducing these risks. Stroke is now the fifth leading cause of death in the nation and a major cause of disability in adults. Stroke is a disease that affects the arteries leading to the brain, or arteries within the brain. According to the National Institute of Neurological Disorders and Stroke (NINDS), an arm of the National Institutes of Health, stroke occurs when there is a sudden interruption in blood supply to the brain. Or when a blood vessel within the brain busts and spills its blood onto brain cells. Since brain cells cannot survive without oxygen and nutrients carried by the blood, they die.

There are two kinds of stroke: ischemic stroke (blockage of blood vessels supplying food and oxygen to the brain) and hemorrhagic stroke (bleeding in the brain). Common symptoms of stroke include "sudden numbness or weakness, especially on one side of the body; sudden confusion or trouble speaking or understanding speech; sudden trouble seeing in one or both eyes; sudden trouble with walking, dizziness, or loss of balance or coordination; or sudden severe headache with no known cause."[44] According to the American Stroke Association, about 795,000 Americans each year suffer a new or recurrent stroke, with more than 129,000 deaths per year resulting from stroke.[45]

So, is there any evidence that fasting may reduce the risk of stroke or increase the odds of surviving a stroke? A number of studies suggest this is true. Perhaps the most important way fasting protects against stroke is the role it plays in preserving a healthy cardiovascular system and regulating blood pressure.

In a major clinical human trial conducted in the United States and published in the *Proceedings of the National Academy of Science* in 2011, doctors showed that people on a calorie reduction demonstrated reduction in well-known risk factors for ischemic stroke such as body fat, blood pressure, and serum lipid and lipoprotein levels. In that study researchers placed eighteen individuals on calorie reduction for about seven years, with a control group of another eighteen age-matched healthy individuals following a typical American diet. The researchers measured several biomarkers of cardiovascular disease, such as serum lipids and lipoproteins, fasting plasma glucose and insulin, blood pressure, high-sensitivity C-reactive protein, and body composition. At the end of seven years the fasting group showed normalized blood pressure. In addition, all the other factors for cardiovascular risks were higher in those who ate normal diets than for those who fasted.[46]

Simply put, this study showed convincingly that fasting reduces the risk of atherosclerosis, a condition closely linked to stroke. In fact, in another study researchers showed that BDNF and other neurotrophic factors were upregulated for fasting mice after experiencing ischemic stroke.[47]

So, does fasting protect in some ways against stroke or at least reduce the risk? Studies suggest it does. Human studies are still scarce, but we seem to have enough studies already accumulated in this area to take the outcomes seriously.

Part 2

FASTING FOR THE WHOLE PERSON

Chapter 9

HEALTH BENEFITS OF CHRISTIAN FASTING

Fasting possesses great power. If practiced with the
right intention, it makes one a friend of God.

—QUINTUS TERTULLIAN (AD 160–220)
EARLY CHURCH LEADER AND AUTHOR[1]

S<small>O FAR</small> I <small>HAVE EXAMINED GENERAL SCIENTIFIC</small>
information regarding fasting without specific men-
tion of religion. Still, it is worth examining whether
fasting has any beneficial health effects for those who fast
for spiritual purposes. Although there are many types of
fasting within Christendom, in this chapter I will focus on
those for which published, peer-reviewed scientific studies
exist. For the purpose of this discussion, I will group them
into two major categories: the Daniel fast and Lenten (and
other Greek Orthodox) fasts.

The Daniel fast

The Daniel fast is a common practice within many Christian circles. The length of such fasts can vary. This type is named after the story of two fasts followed by the Old Testament prophet Daniel (Dan. 1:8–14; 10:2–3). In the first—and most familiar to Christians—Daniel requested that he and his three Hebrew friends be provided only vegetables to eat and water to drink for ten days. They chose this strict diet instead of partaking of (and defiling themselves with) the royal food and wine provided at the palace. Here is a short account of this event from the Bible:

> Daniel then said to the guard whom the chief official had appointed over Daniel, Hananiah, Mishael and Azariah, "Please test your servants for ten days: Give us nothing but vegetables to eat and water to drink. Then compare our appearance with that of the young men who eat the royal food, and treat your servants in accordance with what you see." So he agreed to this and tested them for ten days.
>
> At the end of the ten days they looked healthier and better nourished than any of the young men who ate the royal food. So the guard took away their choice food and the wine they were to drink and gave them vegetables instead.
>
> —Daniel 1:11–16, niv

Interestingly at the end of ten days Daniel and his friends "looked healthier and better nourished" than others who ate sumptuous meals provided by the king. Could there be any scientific basis to this observation? Fortunately a few studies have measured specific health markers in people going through the Daniel fast in modern times.

As though encouraged by his initial success, Daniel later reported fasting for twenty-one days during which "I ate no choice food; no meat or wine touched my lips; and I used no lotions at all until the three weeks were over" (Dan. 10:3, NIV).

Connecting both versions, modern observances cover a certain period (usually ten, twenty-one, or forty days) in which a Christian abstains from meat and dairy products and eats only vegetables, fruits, whole grains, nuts, seeds, and oils. The primary purpose is to restrict food intake while focusing on prayer and consecration. In this regard, a Daniel Fast meal resembles a vegetarian diet. However, it is even stricter because it includes avoiding alcohol, coffee, food preservatives, sweeteners, additives, and flavors. Indeed, the Daniel fast is a form of dietary restriction, as opposed to a program of caloric restriction. Bear that in mind as I examine some of its health benefits.

A scientific survey

Dr. Richard Bloomer, director of the Cardiorespiratory/ Metabolic Laboratory at The University of Memphis in Tennessee, and his colleagues have published the most studies in this area. They include a 2010 article reporting on the effects of a twenty-one day Daniel fast on metabolic and cardiovascular disease risk factors. Their investigation of health biomarkers included forty-three people (thirteen men and thirty women, 35 ± 1 years; range: 20–62 years) who followed a diet of vegetables, fruits, and nuts. Participants followed detailed guidelines and met periodically with investigators. (It is important to note that these individuals purchased their own foods.)[2]

On the first day of the fast participants reported to the lab for a physical examination, with investigators drawing blood samples for a thorough screening of biological markers for cardiovascular and metabolic risks. At the end of the fast participants again had blood samples drawn for screening. Before both visits participants followed a twelve-hour fasting routine and did not perform any strenuous physical activity or exercise during the preceding twenty-four to forty-eight hours. Researchers measured an extensive set of mental and physical health variables. They included resting heart rate, blood pressure, blood count, a metabolic panel, a lipid panel, and insulin. Researchers also evaluated a homeostatic model assessment, to measure insulin resistance; and C-reactive protein, to determine inflammation and tendency to develop coronary artery disease.

The first thing the study revealed: the spiritual motivation for fasting significantly improved compliance with the fast. I will discuss this spiritual element shortly, but will note here that fasting with the goal of drawing closer to God in prayer and meditation is a crucial factor in seeing benefits from fasting. For this particular study participants' compliance rate was 98.7 percent.

The next important revelation came from the fact that all the biological markers measured for cardiovascular and metabolic health risks significantly ($P < 0.05$) improved among the participants by the end of the study. Specifically they showed marked reductions in total and LDL cholesterol (the bad kind) and systolic and diastolic blood pressure, and important (though not scientifically significant) reductions in insulin, HOMA-IR, and C-reactive protein.[3]

So, in simple language what does this all mean? A key finding is how this study shows that the Daniel fast can lower the risk of developing heart disease and insulin resistance, the latter directly related to diabetes. Another major highlight is how the Daniel fast helped reduce the level of radicals and reactive oxygen species—chemicals such as malondialdehyde (MDA), hydrogen peroxide (H_2O_2), and nitrate/nitrite (NOx), which cause oxidative damage to DNA.[4] These latter findings were published in a 2011 report. Another benefit that emerged from the latter study involved participants reporting improved mood at the end and expressing the desire to continue this kind of fast on their own.

More to the story

The researchers observed a slight downside, however, that is worth mentioning—namely, a significant reduction in total cholesterol. Now, that is a positive in relation to reducing the risk of clogged arteries; lower LDL ("bad" cholesterol) spells lower risks for the heart. However, because there was a dramatic reduction in total cholesterol, it also means that there was a reduction in HDL, or "good" cholesterol.

To understand why this is important, I need to offer a quick explanation of these two types of cholesterol. While the American Heart Association has a simple, easy-to-follow guide on its website,[5] I will summarize. Since cholesterol cannot dissolve in the blood, it needs to be carried to and from body cells by special biological "taxis," called transporters. In this case there are two kinds of "taxi cabs" available—low-density lipoproteins (LDL) and high-density lipoproteins (HDL). As it turns out, the LDL does a lousy job of carrying cholesterol and instead accumulates in blood vessels, where it forms plaques. These plaques can eventually block arteries and cause a range of serious diseases such as heart attack and stroke. So, it's a bad thing when there are more of these LDL cholesterols available.

On the other hand, the high-density lipoproteins help in ridding the bloodstream of those bad LDL cholesterols. It is believed that HDL cholesterol carries off the LDL cholesterol to the liver, where the body breaks down LDL and eliminates it from the system. So, a relatively high level of HDL cholesterol is considered good for cardiovascular health. It is therefore important to not only have a low level of LDL, but also a high level of HDL.

This means that the fact that HDL cholesterol was lowered in participants in the Daniel fast is significant. Fortunately the reason for this is obvious and can be fixed. Because of the nature of the Daniel fast, natural sources of HDL cholesterol (such as lean meat) are eliminated. Hopefully these results can be adjusted by introducing certain sources of HDL cholesterol into the Daniel fast diet, in order to determine whether this corrects the problem. Indeed, a follow-up study examined this very issue.[6]

Published in 2013, the study involved twenty-nine individuals. Sixteen followed the traditional Daniel fast diet, and thirteen did a slightly modified version. The modification introduced one serving of lean meat or skim milk daily to supply natural sources of HDL cholesterol. Again, the compliance rate was high and comparable between the two groups, with the traditional showing a slightly higher compliance rate (96.0 ± 0.94 percent versus 91.4 ± 3.1 percent for the modified group).

The study again showed improvement in reduction of risk factors for cardiovascular disease for both groups, in terms of reduction of total cholesterol. In relation to HDL cholesterol levels for the two groups, the traditional Daniel fast group saw more reduction (13.3 percent) in comparison to the modified group (7.6 percent). Granted, the difference between the two groups in regard to HDL is not statistically significant. Still, considering the relatively small sample size involved, the difference between these two is important.

What is the practical relevance? Both studies show that while the Daniel fast is beneficial to cardiovascular and metabolic health, you need to be intentional in including natural sources of HDL in your diet during a Daniel fast, especially if you plan to make it part of an ongoing lifestyle. Some natural sources of HDL cholesterol include lean meat (avoid meat with fat that can cause additional problems), skim milk, fish (salmon or tuna), avocados, nuts, peanut butter, flax seeds, and olive oil. Physical activity and exercise and weight loss will also boost your HDL level.

Lenten fasts

Another form of Christian fasting investigated scientifically for its role on human health is fasts for Lent and related Greek Orthodox occasions. For many Christians, the forty-eight days before Easter are usually a time to engage in dietary restrictions. Often, during this period— known as Lent—many Christians abstain from dairy products, meat, and eggs. They may use olive oil on week-ends, and fish is only allowed on March 25 and on Palm Sunday, which is a week before Easter. Greek Orthodox Christians practice a similar fast during the forty days before Christmas.

Both types of fasting are similar, and studies on both also report similar results. In general, studies on Lent and other Greek Orthodox fasts show that they lower total cholesterol, as well as LDL cholesterol, which is good for the heart. However, the effects of this fasting on blood pressure and other health indicators are either inconclusive or conflicting. For example, while one study showed that the blood pressure for participants dropped, another study did not find a significant difference between the blood pressure of fasters and non-fasters.[7] Therefore, more studies of this type of religious fasting need to be completed.

Chapter 10

FASTING FOR
TOTAL WELL-BEING

*Dear friend, I pray that you may enjoy good health and that all
may go well with you, even as your soul is getting along well.*

—3 John 2, niv

F AST WITH THE AIM OF IMPROVING THE WHOLE SELF.
In the first half of this book I reviewed the immense
benefits of fasting on human health, mostly as it
relates to body and mind. But, aside from the Christian
fasts I examined in the previous chapter, are there some
spiritual benefits to fasting? As it turns out, the answer is a
resounding "yes!" This is why I started shifting in the previous chapter from looking at physical studies of fasting
to a more holistic view that encompasses spirit, soul, and
body. In the second half of this book my emphasis will
be the implications of fasting for the health of the inner
person—and therefore the whole person.

In the preceding chapter I examined the role of religious fasting on human health. While these scientific studies are preliminary, they found similar improvements in health biomarkers, which I reviewed in the first eight chapters. As I mentioned, these studies found increased compliance from the participants, chiefly because their major goal in fasting was spiritual. Purpose is a powerful force, a topic I addressed in an earlier book, *The Search for Meaning: Living for a Higher Purpose.* When your focus shifts from merely losing weight to maintaining a healthy spiritual, physical, and mental balance, you will reap immense benefits from fasting. There is something about fasting that helps develop moderation, instills self-discipline, and affects not only the body but also the spirit, giving it the opportunity to self-renew.

It is no wonder that John prayed that his friend Gaius would live in good health. The powerful health benefits of fasting for the human body ought to get your attention. Good health is certainly an important goal for everyone. That health involves both the mind and the body. It is the true picture of wellness: a healthy and fulfilling life. This is the kind of life in which health span is improved for the body and mind, and the person is enabled to enjoy a prosperous spiritual life. This is total well-being that affects body, mind (or soul), and spirit. There is no escaping it—to feel truly fulfilled in this world we live in, we not only have to take care of the body, but we must also take care of our mental and spiritual health. When we neglect any one of those three aspects, our lives tilt out of balance. Fortunately fasting impacts all three aspects positively.

To focus exclusively on physical health benefits is to glimpse a limited picture. Fasting has been practiced for centuries, mostly for spiritual reasons. There are good reasons for that, as you shall see in the chapters that follow. It is only in recent times that the physical health benefits have come to our attention. As wonderful as those health benefits are, they cannot supplant fasting's spiritual benefits. Clearly the spiritual and health gains from fasting are complementary and mutually beneficial.

A human being is essentially spirit, has a soul (mind, will, and emotions), and lives in a body. Our body is the "house" in which we live and exercise our being on this planet Earth. While it is true that fasting impacts primarily the human "house," this primary benefit translates to other benefits for the soul and spirit. When the body is healthy, the rest of the three-part being is able to function freely. Also, during times of fasting we train our inner being to refrain, choose discipline, refuse overindulgence, and celebrate a life that goes deeper than food, drink, and material existence.

Fasting goals

Given the spiritual basis of fasting, it is important to fast with both spiritual and physical goals in mind. Shortly I will provide some practical suggestions about different kinds of fasts you can follow. Still, it is up to you to choose a fasting program that works for you. It may be the Daniel fast, where you dedicate about twenty-one days to a partial fast that features mainly fruits and vegetables. Or you may choose to fast and renew yourself for a day—or two or three—a week. Or you may cut back 20 percent or so of your daily energy intake and live a "fasted lifestyle."

Whichever practice you choose, you need to see this season as a time to renew the whole person. Such days of fasting can present a huge opportunity to read a book, pray, meditate and draw closer to God, reevaluate the path you are on in life, intercede for a hurting friend and a broken world, or lend a helping hand to building your community. After all, fasting teaches us to cut back a bit on indulging self and make life a little less about us. In this sense, fasting can help us see the big picture about life.

If you are only concerned about weight loss and looks, you may lose an amazing opportunity to tap into a huge aspect of fasting that has benefited generations past. For sure, looking good and feeling good is important. However, being healthy physically, spiritually, and mentally is ultimately the most important issue. Life is certainly more than our appearance. You are likely to become exhausted if your main goal is to lose weight and look good. Past scientific studies have shown that people who are overly concerned about their weight are more likely to develop eating disorders.[1]

Eating disorders

There are a number of eating disorders: anorexia nervosa, bulimia nervosa, binge eating disorder, and orthorexia nervosa. Like every good thing, calorie restriction (fasting) can be abused, which can lead to disorders. While people with orthorexia nervosa become excessively preoccupied with avoiding food considered unhealthy, individuals with anorexia nervosa are so preoccupied with losing weight that they end up losing far too much. On the other hand, fanatical alternate day or intermittent fasting can lead to development of bulimia nervosa or binge eating disorder (usually after fasting). Moderation is a virtue. Accept your freedom from fads and the transient opinions of others. Instead, embark on a fasting and calorie-restricted journey that is right for you.

Understanding your identity as a spiritual being brings freedom from excessive fear of gaining weight and losing your good looks. Fasting will help you lose weight, but I have intentionally not highlighted that aspect because of the tendency to turn fasting into just another weight-loss program. In fact, in some cases individuals who are already too concerned about their weight and physical appearance may develop anorexia after a prolonged fasting program. On the other hand, calorie restriction (fasting) can indeed be a cure for anorexia when there is an emphasis on the whole person. You are more than your weight. You are spirit, you have a soul, and you live in this "house" called a body. Accept the immeasurable worth of the real you.

For sure we ought to be legitimately concerned about excessive weight due to the fact that it increases the risk for certain chronic diseases such as diabetes, heart disease, stroke, and high blood pressure. But one can become unduly concerned about weight. We can define ourselves and people around us by our BMI (body mass index) reading. There is much more to a person than his or her weight. At the end of the day the essence of our being isn't merely physical, but spiritual.

On the other spectrum of anorexia are two other eating disorders known as bulimia nervosa and binge eating disorder. What these two disorders have in common is the tendency (sometimes uncontrollable) to overeat and gorge oneself. While bulimia nervosa follows the episode of excessive eating with purging (usually vomiting), binge eating disorder tends not to do this. Binge eating disorder seems to be the most prevalent eating disorder in the United States. In fact, about 30 percent of those who are overweight suffer from binge eating disorder.

Although fasting can help with such disorders,[2] it is true that some individuals tend to overeat immediately after fasting. So, choosing a fasting program and a tempo that works for you is important. Let moderation guide you. See fasting as a spiritual discipline that enriches your whole being, not a period of painful denial that you are *so looking forward to finishing*. When you train yourself to fast in a way that suits your physiology and style, you won't rush to gorge on food afterward. It gradually becomes a lifestyle and a lifelong habit. When this happens, fasting can become a remedy for binge eating disorders.

My experience has been that when individuals restrict their energy intake with the whole picture in mind—spirit, soul, and body—this higher purpose tends to constrain them from gorging themselves after fasting periods. They know there is a higher purpose for their action. It isn't just self-denial for its own sake. Instead, they view fasting as self-denial that makes the whole person better. This process not only trains the body, but also aligns spirit and soul with eternal principles. This way, fasting isn't seen as a punishment to quickly run away from (in the form of gorging self) at the slightest opportunity, but a celebrated, self-imposed discipline that makes the whole person better.

A sustainable approach

Before discussing various fasting plans, I want to examine how to approach choosing a fasting program that is right for you. It is your responsibility to choose the kind of fasting that works for you in the long run. This is what I call fasting for life: the kind of lifestyle that is both sustainable and beneficial in the long term. Also, by "fasting for life," I mean fasting in such a way that you experience fullness of life, complete wellness, and the "all-may-go-well-with-you" kind of life John wrote about. Resist the temptation to become obsessed with one component of the various blessings of fasting.

Fasting can be useful for improving health span and reducing our risk of such chronic diseases as diabetes, cancer, and neurodegenerative diseases. But fasting is also a powerful spiritual tool that helps us stay in tune with God and enjoy a full, balanced life. Both aspects of fasting are important, but in my opinion to shift focus from spiritual to solely health will be a mistake. Fasting will help you lose weight; in almost all the studies referenced in the first section, nearly all the subjects involved in each study did so. However, to refocus fasting efforts just to lose weight is, to say the least, myopic. Fast in such a way that you maximize fasting's health, mental, and spiritual benefits. After all, it is all about attitude, which is why you must choose a sustainable plan. Don't become too ambitious and decide to fast for forty days when you have not yet done two days.

Take it one step at a time. Start now to cut back on your calorie intake and to intentionally fast from time to time, but avoid going to extremes.

There is a good reason for describing fasting as a "discipline." Every discipline requires training, practice, consistency, and a measure of sacrifice. Fasting is a spiritual sacrifice, one that is self-imposed. There is a cost—denying yourself food at a regular rate is not going to be a lot of fun. This is probably why many people don't fast; it takes discipline. You have to choose to make this sacrifice.

This is important because some people may read about these benefits of fasting discussed earlier and feel motivated enough to fast periodically. That is a wonderful thing. But you have to realize that fasting is in some ways a painful practice, and mentally commit to do it anyway. I think the initial sacrifice involved in fasting seems to come as something of a shock to people who are just starting. Often, this initial pain results in the discontinuation of the program. Whenever you start a fast, your body will likely go into a kind of "revolt." Denying it a constant supply of food and chemicals is too much of a sacrifice, leaving you feeling weak, tired, and maybe even dizzy. But as everyone who fasts can tell you, that all-consuming feeling of pain and weakness gets better as you persist.

Remember, biomedical scientists view fasting as a biological stressor—such initial reactions are a result of this mild biological stress. However, as you persevere, your body sets in motion a range of biochemical processes to counter this new "stress." Recall that it is this hormetic effect that makes fasting so beneficial.

So, what is the point? Fasting involves a cost, so accept this fact firmly before choosing to fast. Then persevere. In this initial stress-hormesis phase, it is also important to choose a plan that gradually increases in length and intensity. For example, if you haven't fasted for a long time, start with skipping breakfast; fast until noon. After a while, skip breakfast and lunch, and eat a normal meal in the evening—and so on.

Training and practice

Training and practice are important elements of a disciplined life. It takes a while for your body to be trained to adjust to the stress of fasting, and to expect it. This is called "conditioning." However, this training won't occur without the regular practice of fasting. In the peer-reviewed, published studies I examined, researchers found fasting is often more beneficial if the compliance level is very high over a relatively long period of time. In other words, if fasting is going to be beneficial to you, spiritually and health-wise, then you have to make a practice of it. Consistency is vital. If you are fasting once a week, say on Wednesdays from morning until night, make this an ongoing routine. After a while your body will "expect" this "stress." It grows conditioned to release hormetic processes that turn out to be beneficial in the long run. This is why you must train yourself to be consistent regardless of the fasting plan you choose.

Furthermore, your choice of fasting program must be guided by sustainability. Ask yourself, "Can I sustain this plan at this stage of my life?" Don't choose a fast just to make an impression, whether on yourself or on others. It is futile to choose a fast that you cannot maintain or sustain. Life is a journey, so the fasting that is right for you today may not work tomorrow in another season of life. Likewise, just because you did certain kinds of fasts in the past does not mean you shouldn't explore other options that are more fitting for you today.

Of course, you are free to try any plan or combination of plans that works for you at any given period. After all, it's your life, so you should enjoy the fasting experiment. Don't beat yourself up if you fail with a particular plan. Try again and choose a different one, or make up your own. As long as you are intentionally working on cutting down calorie intake, you are doing great. This is not a dieting fad to get worked up about. This is fasting for the long haul. It is OK to falter once in a while. This is hoping that every step you take in this journey represents a celebrated "arrival."

Finally, remember that the scientific definition of fasting is simply cutting your total energy intake by 20 to 40 percent without incurring malnutrition. While spiritual fasting may take different forms, it is important to bear in mind that your body can only sustain a certain amount of stress. There is a limit to hormesis, which means you must listen to your body. If you cut your energy intake too much too quickly, fasting may end up being a disadvantage. There is only so much stress the biological system can endure, after which hormetic benefits reach a point of diminishing returns.

You have to be wise about choosing a fasting type. I know that some church groups can become legalistic about fasting. Those who fall into this trap all but mandate that members follow a certain kind of fast *no matter what*. Such rigidity does not effectively give room for grace and flexibility. What this does is place a certain amount of guilt on folks that unless they do *exactly* the fast their church demands and how it demands it, they are doing something wrong and therefore will not be blessed. Biomedically speaking, this kind of attitude is dangerous. While some members can absorb several days of fasting and still be OK, that may not be appropriate for everyone. A better approach to corporate fasting is to state the group's fasting goals. Then, show members enough grace and flexibility to experience the joy of fasting and praying together, even if they don't meet certain guidelines.

Chapter 11

DIFFERENT PLANS

The purpose of fasting is to loosen to some degree the ties which bind us to the world of material things and our surroundings as a whole, in order that we may concentrate all our spiritual powers upon the unseen and eternal things.

—Ole Hallesby (1872–1961)
Norwegian author and theologian[1]

Fasting is abstaining from anything that hinders prayer.

—Andrew Bonar (1810–1892)
Leader in Scottish revival[2]

ALTHOUGH I HAVE DISCUSSED THE NEED FOR organizing a sustainable fast designed for your lifestyle, many readers may still wonder, "How? When? What kind of practical fasting plans are available?" In this chapter I will review some common fasting programs. Keep in mind the kind that incorporates prayer and spiritual development. No matter what type you choose, make prayer and meditation an integral part of it. Following is a menu of possibilities. You may start with one and move to the next. Or you could try different plans to see which one works best for you.

Plan A: Sustained reduced energy intake

This approach involves cutting daily energy intake by 20 percent. After a sustained period—say two to three months—cut back further, to 30 percent. See how long you can sustain this approach. If after a few months you feel like increasing your energy intake slightly, that is fine (you live to fight another day, so to speak). Remember, this is a lifestyle. You may choose a more modest, incremental plan. Say, start with a 10 percent reduction, and then increase to 15 percent, 20 percent, and so on.

Still, when we have followed a fasting program at our church, many people raise such questions as, "What exactly do I need to cut off in order to achieve a 30 percent calorie restriction?" or "How do I calculate my calorie intake?" A quick online search will reveal several calorie calculators that are handy for daily use. Yet I caution against using them as a strict guide; each person is different. In addition, most of these were designed as weight-loss calculators. Plus, not every person has the same energy needs. Indeed, your energy needs will vary from time to time, depending on such factors as the stress of a major deadline project at work, or energy expenditure for a home improvement project.

However, the kind of fasting I advocate is a holistic, life-long plan. You know how much you exercise, how much you eat, how often you eat, and how much snacking you do between meals. This is about you, so keep it simple—the simpler it is to follow, the more likely you are to stick with it. Cut back about 20 percent of current consumption, and go from there. That won't take a scientific calculator. After all, most calorie calculations don't last a lifetime. A habit as simple as checking the total calorie label on food packages will reveal a lot about your calorie intake.

The key to any plan is portion control. For example, start by cutting the size of the portions you eat at each meal by 20 percent. If you still seek some calorie guidelines, recognize that on average, a healthy person's daily calorie requirement tends to be about ten to twelve times his or her body weight. For example, if you weigh 180 pounds, your calorie intake should fall between 1,800 and 2,160 calories per day. If you consider that the average sixteen-ounce sugary drink contains about 210 calories, that is roughly 10 to 13 percent of your daily caloric load.

Plan B: Alternate-day fasting

There are two kinds of alternate-day fasting.

For the first kind, choose one day in the week to do a partial fasting: skip breakfast and lunch and then eat dinner. Say you choose to fast on Mondays and eat as you would normally on Tuesday. Then, on Wednesday and Thursday, repeat the cycle.

Another type of alternate-day fasting is to go a full day without food, drinking only water. In other words, don't eat from Monday morning until you break the fast on Tuesday morning and eat regular meals that day. On Wednesday, you start the cycle again. The advantage of alternate-day fasting is that, as studies I have already examined show, it offers significant health benefits. Also, this kind of fasting is useful when you want to incorporate prayer and spiritual meditation into the fasting period—it allows you enough time of separation and concentration to focus on prayer. The downside is the inability to sustain this kind of fasting for life. Most people who do this tend to do it for a season and then move on to other more sustainable forms.

Plan C: Intermittent fasting

Due to the challenges of maintaining alternate-day fasting for a long period of time, intermittent fasting tends to be the preferred form for many people, including Christians. Intermittent fasting means fasting intermittently but consistently. The most common version of this is fasting on certain days (on Wednesdays and Fridays, for example) while eating normal meals every other day. Some people choose Fridays and Sundays because of the opportunity the weekend offers to slow down and spiritually renew. Again, individual circumstances vary. Fasting Mondays and Fridays may work for you; it could be Tuesdays and Thursdays. Make it *your* plan. It doesn't matter the day (or days) you choose, since you have to base your choice on convenience and functionality.

Follow this two-day partial fasting plan for as long as you are able; it may be for years. Then, if possible, increase to three alternate days in the week. If this approach works for you, make it permanent. I know some people who have trained themselves to fast twice a week consistently. But there is not any kind of "law" about this. In other words, if you skip a week here or there because of circumstances, holidays, or a vacation, the world won't end. The goal is consistency, not perfection. Just keep at it.

If you are new to this discipline, choose a day to start when you may be relatively free and are able to slow down and allow your body to adjust to the stress. Choosing to start your fast on a day that you are facing work pressures or other deadlines may pose more of a challenge than you imagine.

Plan D: Partial multiday fast

Partial multiday fasting involves eating only dinner and skipping breakfast and lunch for several days at a time. Often, this involves a three-day or a seven-day fast, or even longer. In scientific terms this qualifies as intense calorie restriction. Many Christians adopt this kind of fasting, especially when they choose to give themselves to prayer and meditation. This fast offers ample time to receive divine wisdom and grace.

However, this fast is best engaged when you have time to be away from work or other strenuous activities. For many people, this may be during a long weekend, such as a Saturday-through-Monday holiday time frame. I suggest that you *not start* with this kind if you are new to fasting. It is often better to graduate to this kind after practicing intermittent or alternate-day fasting. During this kind of multiday fast, you should drink lots of water to stay well hydrated (forget what you may have heard about abstaining from even water to follow a "pure" fasting routine).

Plan E: Complete multiday fast

Complete multiday fasting includes everything involved in partial multiday fasting, except there is no food whatsoever. Not even fruits, nuts, or vegetables; this is a plan of complete calorie restriction. This is what some people call "dry fasting," except that you should stay hydrated by drinking water. Most people who follow this plan tend to do this for three to seven days. This is not for the faint of heart. Even in Scripture people engaged in this kind of fast only when they were desperate and devoted all their time to seeking God in prayer. Examples are the nation of Nineveh after Jonah warned of God's judgment (Jon. 3:1–10), or Israel after the armies of Ammon, Moab, and Mount Seir threatened to wipe them off the face of the earth (2 Chron. 20:1–4).

I have found that this kind of fasting is practiced more in developing countries than in the United States. Your hunger for God or for His supernatural intervention has to be so intense as to engage fully with God. It is a fast that screams, "God, I need Your help more than words can express!" This is a fast that is devoted to prayer, quietness, and spiritual renewal. It is a kind of fasting you do when you are on a retreat, away from life's noisy chatter and distractions. Minimize activity when doing this fast, and drink water often.

I certainly do not recommend you attempt this kind of fast unless you have followed other less-demanding kinds. If you are going to go beyond three days, I recommend first consulting with either your doctor or someone who is experienced in fasting. Studies suggest that this kind of intense calorie restriction has a far greater hormetic effect on the body, usually in the days after the fast itself. Of course, the disadvantage is the difficulty involved in going for several days without food, which is why relatively few people do this kind.

Plan F: Fruit and vegetable fast

Fruit-and-vegetable fasts are becoming more popular. Not only does this type of fast supply needed nutrients, but also the compliance rates are much higher. There are several kinds of these types of fast, but their common theme is feeding only on fruits and vegetables for a certain period of time. A fruit fast can be for one day or several days at a time. You can embark on a partial or full fast. A partial kind includes eating only fruits and vegetables for breakfast and lunch, and then a full meal for dinner. This is often the most convenient form of fasting for beginners. It is a good way to train your body to let go of its cravings for food and chemicals. However, you can choose to do a complete fast, which means nothing but fruits and vegetables throughout the fasting period. Scientifically speaking, for a fruit fast to have the same effect as chronic caloric restriction (such as a three-day complete fast), it needs to be prolonged. Whether it is partial or complete, sustaining a fruit fast for a relatively longer period gives the body enough time to kick into hormetic mode. This is why the more common versions of fruit and vegetable fasts are often for seven, ten, twenty-one, or forty days.

When this fasting lasts for a minimum of twenty-one days, it is popularly known as a Daniel fast, which I discussed previously. As with any method, you should adapt this to your schedule and lifestyle. For example, you could start with three consecutive days in a month when you eat nothing but fruits and vegetables, and drink lots of water. Then you may graduate to doing this for a whole week once a quarter.

Another thing to note about fruit fasts: you need to be intentional about including sources of good HDL cholesterol. In previous studies of Christian fasting fruit fasts proved consistently deficient in this characteristic; it tends to reduce total levels of cholesterol and triglycerides. While that is good, the downside is how it tends to also lower the supply of the HDL cholesterol. A good way to counteract this is by including some nuts; peanuts, walnuts, and cashew nuts are rich sources of HDL cholesterol. Another good source is olive oil.

Water and fasting

Should you drink water while you fast? Yes, yes, and yes. When I first started fasting several years ago, several people told me that in order to do complete, "dry fasting," I shouldn't drink any water. So, in those days I embarked on three or more days of complete fasting without a drop of liquid nourishment. Bad idea, since that is not healthy. Fasting is a spiritual discipline, not an exercise in spiritual recklessness. Your body needs water to survive; for the average adult, water constitutes between 50 and 65 percent of body mass. Water is the main solvent for most solutes and chemicals in the body. Also, water maintains a good temperature balance within the body.

This begs the question: why would we deny the body water during a period of significant stress? Besides, staying adequately hydrated during fasting helps with the detoxification process as the body excretes toxins through urine and sweat. After all, we are not fasting to earn God's blessings. Fasting helps to condition us to receive from God and to renew spirit, soul, and body. So, the idea that drinking water is somehow equivalent to eating and therefore reduces the effect of fasting is at best born out of human self-righteousness—in other words, what the Scriptures sometimes refer to as the "arm of flesh."

Breaking your fast

How do you break a fast, especially a complete fast or prolonged fruit fast? Start with fluids, such as a cup of juice. Also, introduce soft food, such as custard or yogurt. Then, slowly introduce solid food. Whatever you do, go easy on your food intake after fasting. Rushing your body with lots of solid foods after a fast may create shock to the system and result in stomach irritation and/or constipation. You need to gradually retrain your body to come off the stress-hormesis mode it entered during fasting. Balance and moderation is the key.

One constant temptation after a fast is to gorge on food and choose oversized portions. Resist this temptation! It goes to the heart of the discipline fasting is meant to help instill. Let your moderation be made known—to yourself—after fasting, and slowly increase portion size over a period of time until you return to your regular portion.

Chapter 12

FASTING FOR LIFE

I would have lost heart, unless I had believed that I would
see the goodness of the LORD in the land of the living.

—PSALM 27:13, NKJV

Fasting as a religious act increases our sensitivity to that mystery always
and everywhere present to us.... It is an invitation to awareness, a call
to compassion for the needy, a cry of distress, and a song of joy. It is
a discipline of self-restraint, a ritual of purification, and a sanctuary for
offerings of atonement. It is a wellspring for the spiritually dry, a compass
for the spiritually lost, and inner nourishment for the spiritually hungry.

—FATHER THOMAS RYAN, AUTHOR OF *THE SACRED ART OF FASTING*[1]

T IS FASCINATING TO NOTICE A CONDITION THAT SEEMS
to surround discussions of fasting, even from a scientific perspective—the topics of disease, pain, aging, and
depression. In most cases, almost all studies I have referenced show that fasting has some beneficial effects. Still,
fasting in and of itself does not directly cure any disease
or relieve pain. However, it appears to set in motion other

biological "chain reactions" that do have a positive impact on disease or pain.

Therefore, the very idea of fasting calls to mind our humanity, frailty, and mortality. As we age we grow old, develop wrinkles, contract diseases, and eventually die. We ask ourselves, "How could that happen? It seems like it was only yesterday that I looked so young, so healthy, so strong, and so invincible." Life hurtles by so quickly. And while our bodies need food to sustain life, too often in Western cultures—and others around the world that imitate our meat-laden diets—we eat too much and too often. Suddenly that which is meant for our good becomes our undoing. Take chronic obesity, which leaves people at high risk for other chronic diseases. It seems to happen quickly, as one ailment leads to another.

Often left unsaid in the delicate situation of those struggling with overweight conditions is how many people use food to medicate themselves against pain, disappointment, or frustration. One sad event here and a dream that fell apart there can lead to binge eating as a way of escape and dealing with pain. Some habits we develop can serve to make us complacent about life, about our health, and about staying fit. We may shrug, "I'm sure there is still time to work on those. Right now I just want to get through today." Often the pounds add up so slowly that we don't even notice until we are carrying around forty or fifty extra pounds—or more. For many, it seems that we just wake up one day and realize how heavy we have grown. *How* did that happen? *When* did that happen?

In such a situation we can vow to shed some of that weight, only to discover the exercise and other effort involved take a lot of time. Other priorities can make it difficult to concentrate—kids that need to be taken care of, a spouse who needs time, or pressing job responsibilities (after all, that's what puts food on the table). When life overruns us in this way, it seems others like to define us by this extra weight. Friends or family members may make snide remarks and gossip. Society as a whole seems united in its unremitting condemnation or judgment. Sometimes it's not even so much about what is said, but about what is left unsaid. An affirmation denied, a deserved praise not given, or an earned promotion not offered. But this human framework is not our identity. "This weight isn't me," you say. "How can they be so mean? If only they knew my story or how hard I have fought to shed these extra pounds. If only I could go back and change a few things."

Land of the living

This less-than-perfect reality of our daily life in community with other people represents what the psalmist called "the land of the living." I think that phrase probably referred to the fact that we live in a defined place and time, and with specific people and circumstances. We live in a particular place, not in a vacuum. We work with colleagues at the workplace, live in a home with spouse and children, worship with others at church, and drive on the same road with other drivers. We live in the land of the living. We are here with others; we are not alone. We suffer not only by the trials and pains we endure, but also by watching and sharing in the pain of those we love.

Likewise, when we are happy, we are also not alone. We have friends and family who rejoice with us when we graduate from high school or college, when we wed, or at the birth of a new child. Even when we depart this world, we usually don't go out alone; we have living relatives and friends who gather to send us on our journey into eternity. We quarrel and make up. We love and occasionally hate. We forgive and are forgiven. We give and receive gifts. Surely we live in the land of the living.

Still, the fact that we live in a fallen world means things can get messy. We are involved with life in all its dimensions and intricacies. The conditions of life in the place where we are may be different from conditions elsewhere. But each of us lives right here, in this place, with these people, at this point in time. We may not have chosen all the people with whom we have to live, but we still have to live a full life wherever we are located. And we can't always control the conditions of our lives, let alone the condition of others in this place. These conditions may change very quickly too.

Take that marriage that started so romantically. You couldn't have been surer that this was the right person for you. When you said, "Yes, I do," you meant it with every fiber of your being and with every iota of joy. You gave it your all too—emotionally, financially, and with all your heart and body. The conditions of this place of marriage seemed so right, so pure, and so divine. Then a few years later you woke up and realized that conditions had changed. *What happened?* Your spouse seemed so invested and so in love; it seems like only yesterday. Today that same spouse seems so disconnected from you. You wonder: "What went wrong? Why the sudden request for a divorce? I thought I addressed those occasional complaints. I thought we were working through our differences. Just when I had mentally and spiritually surrendered myself and my future to this person, I am suddenly facing divorce. How do I get started all over again? This is so unfair."

As unfair as it may seem, millions have lived through the gradual dissolution of the bonds of love. Those ties that birthed a marriage change to bitterness and hatred in the ensuring divorce proceedings and child custody battles. The conditions of this land of the living have changed dramatically. It can sure get messy—precisely because, among other factors, our lives and journey are intricately connected with other people living in this same place.

Alien territory

Thinking of the land of the living, I can't help but view it as this huge, sometimes alien territory that we must navigate during our pilgrimage. We are exploring this land called life. Life itself is a journey. Think of Abraham in search of the land of Canaan and his explorations of the land when he arrived. An exploratory journey like that is packed with excitement. There is the anticipation of what lies ahead, the fulfillment of arriving at the next step in the journey, and the joy of conquering a new land. Yet it is also packed full with challenges—the unexpected, unforeseen circumstances, fear of the unknown, and the danger of arriving at a new place, fresh and vulnerable.

There is no escaping reality. We are going to have our moments of victory, joy, and celebration. We are also going to have times of challenge and testing. There are going to be seasons in life when everything seems to be working so well: the kids are doing well at school, friends recognize your work, and the family is in good health. However, everyone faces transitional seasons in life; those are the times when you haven't quite reached your destination, but you are not in the same place either.

The "in-between" moments are tough. For example, you may have finally started that business you long dreamed about. While everything seems to have taken off, you aren't seeing any profits either. It is one investment after another. These transitional seasons can be hard. You ask, "Should I give up the business now and start something more profitable? Or wait patiently for the investments to slowly bring in profits?" Friends and family are not always very helpful. Indeed, they can be so impatient that you become agitated.

Maybe you don't own a business, but you have invested yourself in your kids. They were everything to you. You worked hard, and saved a lot, and all for their sake. You were glad to do it. Not only was it worth every penny, you would also do it over again in a heartbeat. But now they are grown up and about to leave home. You woke up one day and realized that you have not really planned for this day. You gave up your life for their good, but now you have to learn to live again. You have to find a new hobby or a new cause in which to invest. You haven't quite finished working on your new self, but you are no longer the old you. You have derived joy and significance in being a mom or a dad. But now, you ask, "What am I?"

Sometimes we arrive at the end of the journey and find that the destination isn't what it was cracked up to be. We have *worked so hard* to get here, but feel so empty or numb. This graduate degree represented a lifelong goal; now that you have it, it doesn't seem to make much of a lasting difference. Or, as many seniors do, you think about giving your all for so many years and accomplishing so much and changing so many lives while serving God and humanity. Yet you wind up seemingly forgotten, ignored, or wracked with disease. *It doesn't seem fair.* Young people carry on as though you haven't been around that long or don't know that much. Your wisdom seems to be ignored. Your heart is filled with memories and maybe even new dreams, but your body doesn't seem to be able to support active pursuits. All this shows that life's journey is filled with thorns as well as thrills.

The life we have.

Still, this is the life we are given, one that is fraught with uncertainty and often disappointing or disillusioning realities. No wonder David wrote: "I would have lost heart, unless I had believed that I would see the goodness of the LORD in the land of the living" (Ps. 27:13, NKJV). Living in this land requires bravery. We can't lose heart and chicken out. We must live right here, right now, in this place and time, and with all the people with whom we explore this land. We set out exploring this land each day, believing that we will see God's goodness.

After all, we don't refuse to take vacations because we may encounter the unknown, or because of the possibility that the visit may turn out not to be as magnificent as we had imagined.

Meditate on this truth: *God brought you to this place.* He has allowed us to be where we are, with these people. Consequently we must take life by the horns and get about the business of living. We have to believe that there is goodness to be experienced, even in our location. In every season of life we must believe that we can see God's goodness. That is true whether you find yourself in a season of blessing and increase, or in a transitional time when you may question your self-worth, or when you reach the likely end of life and stare eternity in the eye. This land of the living is God's gift to us. Accept it and live intensely and enthusiastically, fully present to God and what He is doing in every corner, wherever you turn.

If you have suffered divorce or the anguish of death, don't refuse to love again because of the fear of pain and disappointment. Instead, invest yourself into the love moments God has given you today. We must all live life to the full, because tomorrow will take care of itself. We hope for His goodness in this new land of love. We can't refuse to have children for fear of how they may turn out tomorrow. After all, none of us can control tomorrow, a fact expressed succinctly by James: "Come now, you who say, 'Today or tomorrow we will go into this city, spend a year there, buy and sell, and make a profit,' whereas you do not know what will happen tomorrow" (James 4:13–14, MEV). Still, we can give our children (or grandchildren) all our love and blessing today and trust God to see the goodness of the Lord in their lives tomorrow. I like the way author and publisher William Feather (1889–1981) put it: "One way to get the most out of life is to look upon it as an adventure."[2]

In speaking about the "goodness of the Lord," David alludes to the fact that there is another sphere of reality that impacts our physical world; namely, that the spiritual life is every bit as important as our physical life. When we appreciate the spiritual dimension of life, God becomes more than a vague, distant concept. When we see Him as a very real person, we take God seriously. David seems to suggest that God is ultimately in control. Some of the trials and circumstances along our path through life may seem thoroughly out of control, but David seemed to believe that God's sovereignty ultimately guided him.

And why not? After all, God knows this land of the living more intimately than any of us. He knew every inch of the land and the conditions of this place long before we arrived. Perhaps He knows something about the "place" that we don't know yet—that we *can* make it. There may be resources available in this location that we can't imagine exist. Still, He knows. Perhaps there are other people whom He has prepared to come alongside us in the new land. How will we find out unless we get there and live the life He chooses for us to live? This is one of the reasons fasting has been practiced for generations. People attuned to spiritual realities seek to condition their bodies and humanity to listen less to self and more to God. He knows what we need and where we are heading. In the place of fasting we quiet down enough to listen to the One with the navigational controls—a kind of celestial GPS.

An activating source

Finally the land of the living implies that "life is the country that Christians live in," as noted author Eugene Peterson puts it.[3] Life: that spiritual quality that makes us human. That hard-to-explain, vital force that keeps us alive, growing, thriving, and exploring this country. Life is that divine ingredient within that endows us with inner strength, hopefulness even in the midst of possible gloom, a sense of wonder, a sense of thankfulness for being human, and a largeness of being that is freeing and exhilarating.

Life is that activating force that wakes us up in the morning, puts a spring into our steps, a song in our hearts, and tears of joy in our eyes. Life is that daily, all-encompassing invitation to embrace not only all that we are, but also all that God is to us. After all, life was God's very first gift to humans at the beginning of time—the first "breath of life," which He breathed into our human progenitor. Life is the vast country we have been called to explore, to enjoy, and to cultivate. Life is that which gives meaning and significance to our "daily-ness" and our ordinariness.

Life is what puts enduring joy and hope within the soul of a woman in labor, a smile on the face of a sacrificing father, and peace for the student toiling through one homework assignment after another. We live our ordinary lives in this land of the living, made worthwhile and livable by that God-given quality called life. When life leaks out of us, then living in this land of the living becomes a chore, a misery, and a struggle. When that happens, we are left with nothing but emptiness and nothingness. When life leaks out, then the daily routines become dreadful and dreaded. Minor irritations take on oversized proportions of pain and anguish. Careless offense and omission by loved ones become life-scarring, unforgivable moments.

Solomon, the wise preacher, described this sad state in this proverb: "A merry heart does good like a medicine, but a broken spirit dries the bones" (Prov. 17:22, MEV). Dry bones are deadly. The bone marrow is where the body regenerates white and red blood cells. It is safe to say that life-regenerating stem cells are also located in the bone marrow. However, this treasure of life within us is clothed with an earthen vessel. Life itself is good and complete, but the vessel in which it is contained isn't leak-proof. The vessel gets old and worn. Over time it develops minor cracks here and there, which are not quickly mended.

These cracks aren't always physical. There are those caused by heartaches, disappointments, loss of loved ones, requests denied, love unrequited, wayward children, and unpleasant or traumatic encounters. There also is the unbridled consumption of food and toxins, substances that damage our vessel. When left unfixed, each crack becomes another minor life-leaking point. Over time these leaking points accumulate and become significant. Sometimes these cracks develop from weariness amid everyday routines. Stay-at-home mothers become worn out, feeling unappreciated and resentful. A teacher becomes disillusioned after years of painful sacrifices that seem to go unnoticed and uncelebrated. A faithful worker becomes embittered after years of being passed over for promotions. A caring pastor becomes cynical after years of indifference (or even betrayal) from parishioners.

Here is the danger: the mom still goes about her duties every day, the teacher still teaches, that worker is still at work as usual, and the pastor is still at church preaching, teaching, and counseling. Yet life has leaked out of their being and therefore out of their service. While schooling, serving, worshipping, eating, and writing go on, they no longer take place in the land of the living.

The value of fasting

Fasting helps us seal these leaks and recover life. Fasting creates a condition in which we are most sensitive to spiritually addressing those life-leaking events that are characterized by pain, scars, disappointment, or excessive toxins. In fasting the spirit gets renewed. So does the physical body. This is why fasting has long been a powerful spiritual discipline practiced by everyone from ancient Jews to early church fathers to current Christians worldwide.

While fasting does not erase life-leaking events, it helps in the spiritual process of sealing them and restoring our inner strength and vitality so we can keep going.

Scientists have proven that fasting can help the physical body to renew and refresh, as I reviewed in the first part of this book. So, imagine the effects fasting can provide for the inner life and the spirit and soul. For the remainder of this book, I will focus on the whole person—especially the role fasting plays on inner wholeness and peace. I'm sure you would agree you want a healthy body. Yet you also should desire wellness in your inner being, which includes peace within and spiritual wholeness. Continue to the next chapter for my discussion of the role of fasting in spiritual renewal.

Chapter 13

FASTING AND SPIRITUAL RENEWAL

For even young people tire and drop out, young folk in their prime stumble and fall. But those who wait upon GOD get fresh strength. They spread their wings and soar like eagles, they run and don't get tired, they walk and don't lag behind.

—ISAIAH 40:30–31

Fasting cleanses the soul, raises the mind, subjects one's flesh to the spirit, renders the heart contrite and humble...

—EARLY CHURCH FATHER SAINT AUGUSTINE (354–430)[1]

Fasting in the biblical sense is choosing not to partake of food because your spiritual hunger is so deep, your determination in intercession so intense, or your spiritual warfare so demanding that you have temporarily set aside even fleshly needs to give yourself to prayer and meditation.

—WESLEY L. DUEWEL, LONGTIME MISSIONARY AND PRAYER LEADER[2]

THE REALITY IS THAT LIFE-LEAKING MOMENTS HAPPEN to all of us. Thousands of years ago the prophet Isaiah wrote that even young people in the prime of life can stumble. The good news is that opportunities for life-renewing moments are also available to everyone. Fasting is one of those life-renewing opportunities that are available for no costs. It gives us a thrilling opportunity to gain fresh strength and spread our wings and soar like eagles. We can run and not tire out in the race of life. We can explore the land of the living without lagging behind. Earlier in his book Isaiah reminded people of their mortality: "All flesh is grass, and all its loveliness is like the flower of the field.... The grass withers, the flower fades, but the word of our God stands forever" (Isa. 40:6, 8, NKJV).

Who among us cannot identify with those words? Life has a way of reminding us of our mortality, whether through fading beauty, increasing wrinkles, graying hair, balding, or the diseases of aging. If natural life is all there is to humanity, that will be depressing. Thankfully there is more to us than our decaying bodies. No wonder the Apostle Paul confidently declared: "So we're not giving up. How could we! Even though on the outside it often looks like things are falling apart on us, on the inside, where God is making new life, not a day goes by without his unfolding grace. These hard times are small potatoes compared to the coming good times, the lavish celebration prepared for us. There's far more here than meets the eye. The things we see now are here today, gone tomorrow. But the things we can't see now will last forever" (2 Cor. 4:16–17).

How can we give up on life when we have an opportunity for inward renewal? Even though on the "outside" things seem to fall apart, on the "inside" God is at work to renew and refresh us. There *is* more to us than frail bodies; we are spirit beings and have souls. The spirit and soul are the inward parts, which defy mortality and live on long after the body decays and dies. The external world may include trials, pains, and difficulties, but with fresh strength within the soul, we can carry on. We can embrace a joyful exploration of the land of the living.

When we fast, we provide God a wonderful opportunity to make life new within. Could this be why the wise preacher wondered aloud: "A healthy spirit conquers adversity, but what can you do when the spirit is crushed?" (Prov. 18:14). A healthy spirit sustains a person in his or her physical infirmities, adversities, and sickness. However, when the person is crushed within, where will he or she summon the strength to overcome the vicissitudes of life? Such a reality shows how renewing the inner person is vital to life's journey.

Dawning of hope

I have always been fascinated by that simple word *but* in the Scriptures. It is an interesting word that negates the previous line of thought and redirects our attention to a new reality. Even youths may fail, *but* those who wait on God can find fresh strength. The body may age and become frail, *but*. A marriage may end up in flames, *but*. Whenever God inserts a *but*, it reverses negativity and brings us hope. He draws us away from the insistent noise of pain and mortality to His divinity within. He sparks in us an openness to the possibility of a new life, the hope of a new beginning, and the possibility of recovery. This rings a note of joy and assurance deep within our souls. Those

FASTING FOR LIFE

who wait on God will get a fresh start, fresh strength, and fresh grace. This begs the question: What does it mean to wait upon the Lord?

The idea of "waiting on the Lord" is central to Christian fasting. This discipline involves letting go of food or other pleasures in order to wait on God. Fasting is therefore an integral part of this wait, but not nearly the whole picture. Fasting provides the right conditions for us to wait on God—a blessed means to a wonderful place of waiting.

No doubt you have been to a good restaurant. From the moment you arrive, someone welcomes you and gets you seated. Another attendant comes along to ask for your food and drink order: "Any appetizers? Sweetened or unsweetened tea? Do you want your steak medium or well-done?" After you are served, the attendant comes along periodically to ask: "Is everything OK? Is there anything else I can get you?"

We know what it means to be waited on—to have someone anticipate our desires and meet them. Waiting on God is a lot like that. During periods of fasting, we make time to wait on the Lord. We extricate ourselves from self-indulgence in order to indulge His presence. We commit to listen and hear what He wants, what He says, and to any instructions He gives. Waiting on God means becoming attentive to God. That is the first and perhaps the most important aspect of that waiting. We ask ourselves: "What is He saying? What is He doing? In the light of what He is saying and doing, what am I doing? Which direction have I been going?"

152

However, as with the restaurant attendant, the point isn't our desires but His: His will, His ways, and His glory. Perhaps this is our greatest need—to pause long enough during our busy rat race to gain a divine perspective and look at the big picture so we can find out what He is doing at this time and in this place. Modern life is hectic; we can easily get so consumed in reaching the destination that we lose sight of the journey itself. We may become so enamored by the challenges of surviving in the land of the living that we do not live the life God wants from us. But the country where we live is designed in such a way that the journey is as important as the final arrival. It is not only the land we are called to explore, it is the life we are living—the very expression of our being, personality, and purpose.

Every step in the land of the living is meant to be in itself an arrival of sorts,[3] a celebration of grace. For example, are you so taken in by the need to provide for the kids that you work so much that you no longer have any time to spend with them and enjoy them as they are growing up? You may wake up one day and discover they are grown up and ready to move on in the world without your input in the areas that matter most, such as character formation, love affirmations, and attentive presence.

The gift of presence

Likewise, fasting gives us an opportunity to be present to the One who is ever present with us—to be present in this place, with the people in this place, and to what God is doing in this phase of our journey. This land of the living is filled to overflowing with God-shaped events,

God-breathed words, God's salvation, God's unexpected provision and recovery, God-arranged "chance" meetings, and God-inspired comeback stories. This land of the living is the land in which God's story is being played out daily. Are we paying any attention to this unfolding story?

It turns out that we are central to this God story. It's God's story, but in many ways it is also the story of God's love and mercy and grace toward us. God wants us to be involved in living out the dynamic story of His love and rescue, even in the midst of a difficult country. During fasting we are forced to quiet down enough to pay attention. When we listen to God during our fast, we can learn enough about what God is doing to become aware of our own role in the plot.

There is also another element of this waiting on God. It involves *attending* to God. During fasting we take a break from "me, I, and mine" to pay attention to Him—to do His will, serve Him and His people, and intently give ourselves and what is ours to Him. When we listen to Him, we gain the wisdom to respond in obedience. In the place of waiting we choose to prioritize our life and our health based on His wisdom. Waiting on God means not only being attentive but also offering a resounding "yes!"

My sense is that an important component of waiting on God is to literally wait *for* God. Indeed, we are so used to today's instant-gratification society that patience has taken on a more significant dimension. Patience has to have its way fully with us—and in us—so that we may grow into the image He has created for us. In the land of waiting on God quick fixes aren't of much help. Life is long and sometimes painstaking. Fasting teaches us to be patient. The only alternative is to take matters into our own hands; many can testify that this didn't quite work out like they hoped.

These days it seems common to hear the stories of husbands and wives who feel shortchanged in their marriage. He prays, talks to his wife, and maybe even attends some counseling sessions with her, mystified by her seeming unhappiness. Meanwhile, the wife wonders, "How can he? I'm making my best effort to address his concerns." He is not happy, but neither is she. Still, they love each other and want to see each other happy. Patience knocks daily at their door, but more often than not, they lock him out.

Finally the husband declares, "I can't take it anymore." He proposes a divorce, and to his surprise, she eagerly agrees. As it turns out, she is also feeling like she can't *live like this* one more minute. They divorce, but when they meet a few months later at a social event, they wonder, *Why did we part from each other? What happened? Did we separate too quickly? Should we have allowed patience more time to do its work?*

Fasting for patience

Waiting is hard for us typically impatient humans, but wait for God we must if we want Him to complete His work of grace in us. Although waiting can indeed be painful, fasting trains us to grow and develop our patience. As the writer of Hebrews said, "But you need to stick it out, staying with God's plan so you'll be there for the promised completion. It won't be long now, he's on the way; he'll show up most any minute. But anyone who is right with me thrives on loyal trust; if he cuts and runs, I won't be very happy. But we're not quitters who lose out. Oh, no! We'll stay with it and survive, trusting all the way" (Heb. 10:36–39).

May I suggest that we stick it out with God's plan until the promised completion? It is tough to endure. Life doesn't always give us what is fair. Yet when we give patience an opportunity to complete its work in us, God is glorified, even in the midst of the challenge. We are called to thrive on loyal trust—trusting God that He will come through. We stay with His plan to the end. In fasting, as tough as this is, we receive the grace to try.

Fasting itself may not be much fun. Our body craves food and nourishment, and rightfully so. But there are immense benefits to the whole being, especially the inner person, that come from fasting. The first is renewed strength. What is this fresh strength? That inner zest to live and keep living; in other words, the courage that comes from the inner being that carries on even when there seems to be no reason to keep going. It is that kind of inner empowerment that Paul prayed that the Ephesians would know: "I pray that out of his glorious riches he may strengthen you with power through his Spirit in your inner being, so that Christ may dwell in your hearts through faith" (Eph. 3:16–17, NIV). This is the kind of strength that comes from God-breathed renewal—a strength that comes from the Holy Spirit, who out of His vast riches of grace imparts some of this grace into our inner being.

Have you ever gone through a season when you felt hunkered down or defeated—maybe on the verge of collapse? It is those times when life-leaking events often occur: the doctor diagnoses a disease, or love given is not returned. At such times the inner person becomes broken and loses the will to carry on. Yet after a while, you find a fresh spark as something happens in your soul to give you a new hope and the courage to start afresh— to keep going, to smile, and to love again. Fasting creates the conditions for God to renew our strength from within, kindle a new fire, and breathe a new life within our souls. As Isaiah said, those who wait on the Lord shall receive fresh strength.

And, as the prophet wrote, when we receive this strength from waiting on the Lord, we shall also spread our wings and soar as eagles. Life is no longer a boring chore to endure. Instead, it becomes an exciting adventure—a daily anticipation of what God will do next. We take each step in hopeful expectation as we turn each corner, knowing that He who knows the end will lead the way. We dare to dream again. In fact, we dream so big now that others who don't understand think we are being presumptuous. We come in good company with the psalmist as we "taste and see that the LORD is good" (Ps. 34:8, NIV). We fall in love again, and go at it with all our heart as though it had never before been broken.

Taking on new meaning

With this kind of outlook, life takes on a new meaning and a new urgency. We learn a new trade, or go back to school. We go to work with a song in our hearts, not because the conditions in the workplace have changed, but because God has given us fresh strength within.

We accept God's love and move on in the world. While the scar of hurt hasn't vanished, we know He holds the future in His hand. Pain has clipped the wings of many who should be soaring as the eagles. Past hurts and disappointments often debilitate otherwise productive people. Yet when we wait on God through fasting and prayer, and receive His fresh grace within, we dust ourselves up from the sad dust of self-pity and despair and take our place in life.

Fasting in God's presence tends to have this kind of impact. This land of the living isn't all it is meant to be without our active participation. Now, we are thankful for this land, for this moment, for this day, for this place. We spread our wings and soar as the eagles.

However, there's more. As Isaiah 40:31 says: "They run and don't get tired, they walk and don't lag behind." I have always wondered why the prophet followed this progression: first, we fly and soar as eagles; then, we run and are not tired; finally, we run and won't lag behind. You would think that we would start off walking, then run, and finally take off flying. Yet when a person has been granted new strength from the riches of God's Spirit, they come out flying. How can we come out of an encounter with God's fresh grace and merely walk? We come out greeting life with a swagger. Do you think that Abraham walked up to his wife and family and nonchalantly told them how God met him and told him to go to a far-off place, where He would bless him and make him a father of many nations? I don't think so! His joy and enthusiasm must have represented the equivalence of soaring as an eagle.

When you first fell in love with your spouse, what was it like? Were you cautious and careful about what others thought about the two of you? I bet you came out swinging at this new way of living and loving with all your energy. You came out soaring as an eagle in this sky of loving and being loved. When you first started that business you had long dreamed about, did you go to work the first day bogged down, cautious and indifferent? I doubt it. I sense that you went to work that day excited and delighted for this opportunity. You were soaring. Being above, in the sky—the challenges of this new life are there, all right; yet to us they don't seem that significant. After all, we are way above them, in the sky. God's renewed grace and opportunity always have that effect on us.

Still, over time those initial feelings of exuberance tend to wear off. We get past the wide-eyed phase and notice the challenges associated with this opportunity; we must *deal with them.* Yet here is the miracle Isaiah talked about—even though we grapple with life's problems, they no longer weary us. We are running now in this rugged land; we are aware of the twists and turns, but we are OK with that. We continue to run the race God has called us to run. While we are not unmindful of the challenges, in spite of them we keep going. Periodic fasting and waiting on God create the conditions for that to happen. We have to continually renew our spirits and bring freshness to our souls. While there is no going around it and no easy way out, we still have pure joy. We are not praying for challenges, but we are ready to step over what the enemy hopes will be a stumbling block. We run and don't get tired, because we have learned to draw from God's strength in the place of fasting and prayer.

Walking to the end

In the final phase of life's journey we are no longer able to fly or run as in younger years. Now, we can only walk. Yet though we walk, we don't lag behind. We are more hesitant now to make bold declarations of faith, but we don't lag behind one bit in trustful obedience. We are no longer cocky or self-assured, but we are even more certain of God's over-reaching grace. We may be considered weak by some, but God's strength is being made ever perfect in us. We may have seen many difficult days and shed many tears, but we have also seen so many "God moments" that we stand in awe of Him.

We don't have as many words as we used to, but our hearts are filled with inexplicable wonder of His glory. As we bow before Him during fasting and prayer, we marvel that He has loved us through these many years, stuck by us, and has done us good. We get up from our knees amazed, grateful for life, and yielded to Him. We may not clap as loud as the younger folk, but our thanksgiving rings just as loud and true. We may not always study the Bible as often and as long as we used to, but we have treasured up His Word in our hearts, so much that in Him we live and love and have our being.

Chapter 14

FASTING AND PRAYER

But this kind does not go out except by prayer and fasting.

—MATTHEW 17:21, MEV

Are any of you suffering hardships? You should pray. Are any of you happy? You should sing praises.... The earnest prayer of a righteous person has great power and produces wonderful results.

—JAMES 5:13, 16, NLT

ASTING AND PRAYER GO TOGETHER. JUST AS FASTING ought to be accompanied by prayer, you should strengthen your prayers with intermittent fasting. The heartfelt prayer of a believing person counts for something in this land of the living. It is effective to meet most of life's challenges. However, as the Lord Jesus reminded His disciples, some challenges can only be conquered through prayer *and* fasting.

Desperate times require fasting and prayer, which is what Jesus told His disciples after they couldn't help a distraught father whose son's epileptic seizures plunged him into fire and water. They prayed and did their best, but were still powerless. The father knew that if no help came, they would have to return home—to danger. It was a desperate situation; having to watch your beloved son suffer and know you can do nothing is pure torture. This kind calls for divine intervention, which is why this desperate dad found his to way to Jesus amid a huge crowd and fell down at His feet to beg for God's mercy. Isn't God's mercy all any of us can reasonably expect? A mercy that includes compassion, grace, forgiveness, and healing. It opens the gate for us to come in to His kindness, salvation, and life, and partake of His riches.

The father's plea didn't go unnoticed. Jesus responded by speaking a word; the devil went out of the boy, and he was cured. Granted, epilepsy may have other underlying biological and physiological causes, but this kind was caused by an evil spirit interfering with this boy's life. It involved spiritual forces at play, beyond mere physical considerations.

There is a spiritual component to human life. We are spirit beings who live in bodies and have souls. We are not merely organic because of the spiritual, intangible aspect of our humanity. Academic literature uses different names, such as the subconscious mind, the metaphysical, or the paranormal. In each of those references a secular culture alludes to an intangible, spiritual element of life. When the spirit realm is connected to God's Spirit, it is influenced by the Holy Spirit and shapes much of our physical existence in a positive way. It bears our infirmities and gives us inner strength to carry on with life victoriously. This gives us a wholesome personality and brings us closer to God.

However, when an evil spirit is allowed to influence our lives, the outcome is often disastrous, leading to hatred, depression, disease, or a broken heart. Since an evil spirit caused this type of epilepsy, the moment Jesus sent that evil spirit away, the boy instantly regained his health. The question is not whether we believe that evil still lurks in this world, but what action we will take when a streak of evil crosses our path.

Desperate seasons

So, what should we do in desperate seasons? Fast and pray and fast. Believing in God's goodness is important, but as the master told His disciples, there may be something else we ought to do when evil touches us physically. There is a great lesson in what happened after Jesus cast out the demon: "Then the disciples came to Jesus privately and said, 'Why could we not cast him out?'" (Matt. 17:19, MEV). The Lord said it was because of their unbelief, and then He told them of the essential nature of prayer and fasting in difficult situations.

When we mix our believing trust in the Lord with fasting and prayer, we intensify our spiritual lives. Desperate times require desperate action. Throughout Scripture, when individuals faced difficult times, they turned to God in prayer while they fasted. I think there is something about including fasting that cries—as Peter did when he feared drowning in the sea—"Lord, save me!" (Matt. 14:30, MEV).

We live in a culture that tells us that we are completely in charge of our lives, and everything we become is what we make of ourselves. While there is a place for taking some responsibility for our lives, you and I know from experience that sometimes desperate moments strike. Sometimes life is out of our control, whether that means a child is diagnosed with cancer, a woman who eats right and exercises faithfully still comes down with cancer, a pastor who serves faithfully for years still sees a child renounce the faith, or an upstanding professional has a child who takes illicit drugs. Instead of growing complacent, times such as these that call for fasting and prayer.

I realize we live in a world that mocks the spiritual and makes caricatures of the idea of pagan worship and evil spirits as if they didn't exist. Yet in your heart you know that evil exists. You may have known close friends whose lives have intersected with evil. In times such as these we must fast and pray to break the influence of evil off their lives. Although not everything that happens to us necessarily has a spiritual root, we know that most things can be dealt with spiritually. If nothing else, praying during fasting helps us to experience God's peace from within: "Don't fret or worry. Instead of worrying, pray. Let petitions and praises shape your worries into prayers, letting God know your concerns. Before you know it, a sense of God's wholeness, everything coming together for good, will come and settle you down. It's wonderful what happens when Christ displaces worry at the center of your life" (Phil. 4:6–7).

David's dilemma

King David found himself in one of those desperate moments during his reign as king of Israel. A series of bad choices caught up with him. First, he committed adultery with the wife of one of his faithful soldiers. Then, when

Bathsheba told him that she was pregnant, he tried to cover up his affair by arranging for the soldier to be brought home, hoping husband and wife would sleep together, as a way of covering up his infidelity. When that didn't work out, he arranged to position Uriah in battle so he would be killed—a diabolical plot that succeeded.

For a while David's conscience must have pricked him. Perhaps he silenced it by promising himself to be a good husband to Bathsheba and a good father to their child. He was determined to *do the right thing* from then on. It is possible to imagine that David calmed his conscience by telling himself that keeping quiet served a "greater good" by maintaining his integrity and ability to rule in peace. After all, bigger things were at stake. There were new battles to fight and enemies to conquer. Why ruin it all because of a "little" mistake? David might have convinced himself, "In the grand scheme of things, isn't the end more important than the means?" So, David took Bathsheba as his wife, and she gave birth to a son. David may have moved on, but God loved him too much to let him off without confronting his sin.

To accomplish the task, God sent the prophet Nathan. After the prophet's rebuke, David genuinely repented. Still, the child grew quite ill. Now, a part of David was irrevocably tied to this baby, who symbolized his resolve to make things right. Naturally he prayed earnestly that the infant would live. The word from Nathan: the baby would eventually die. David prayed otherwise; after all, *he* had sinned, not this poor child. We don't always have answers to life's complicated twists and turns, but an innocent child suffering intensely is too hard for any parent to bear—especially when the parent suspects the child's suffering is due to the parent's past mistakes. David prayed, but the child got sicker. As a result, "David prayed desperately to God for the little boy. He fasted, wouldn't go out, and slept on the floor" (2 Sam. 12:16).

In this desperate moment David not only prayed, but he also fasted. It was his way of saying: "God, this means a lot to me. I am really desperate. Help this child, please!" Notice that as part of the fast, he slept on the floor. The act of sleeping on the floor (instead of his royal bed) as well as putting ashes on his head and renting his clothing were all signs of humility and desperation before God. By these actions, people of old indicated their utter humility and brokenness. In addition, David did not go out. In other words, he gave God the seed of time—time to pray through his pain, time to repent of his sins, time to listen to God, and time to allow God to heal his brokenness. Fasting provides such an opportunity.

I know that we are living in a hectic age where spending time in even a few minutes of prayer is becoming more difficult. To suggest spending extended periods in prayer and fasting seems tenuous at best (even impractical). Yet if we are going to see the God of angel armies intervene in human affairs, we have to offer to God this sacrifice. The act of fasting tells God that we value His intervention strongly enough to commit adequate time to it. Fasting not only intensifies our prayer, but it also clarifies the needs in our lives. But it doesn't force the hand of God. Despite David's fasting, the child didn't live. Still, fasting gives God an opportunity to encounter us, change us, and mold us into His glorious image.

Saying yes to God

When David heard that the boy had died, he got up from his fast, washed up, and dined. He had stayed long enough on his knees to surrender to the almighty God. In fasting he had offered his heart deep enough in the streams of grace to know that if the child died anyway, it must be how the divine heart had willed it. All the ways of God are just; all His works are perfect. He is a God who knows. David knew that he did not just acquiesce to problems and let the devil torment him. He prayed, fasted, and invited God's miracle-working power into his situation. So, bowing his heart in worship, he said yes to God, to His ways, and to His works.

Likewise, when we yield ourselves to God thoroughly—and intensely—in fasting and prayer, we accept His forgiveness and shed our guilt. We know He hears us, that we are beloved to Him, and that His providence protects and provides for us. We can trust His wisdom and power. Sure enough, in the verses that follow, we see a glimpse of God's loving heart toward David. David's fasting, coupled with prayer and repentance, had not been in vain. God was moved by David's posture of repentance and had compassion on him. He promised to give David another son, an heir to his throne, through the same Bathsheba.

Oh, the love and kindness of God. Who can measure the depth of His loving heart? In God's divine economy time spent in fasting and prayer is never wasted. If you look at fasting and prayer as an inefficient use of precious time, you don't understand its value. God wants to spend that time with us so He can heal, save, love, and shape us. Answering our desperate plea for help is part of the equation, but there is more to that plea in God's ears than meets the eye. Sometimes He provides us the physical rescue we cry out for, such as rescuing Israel from the nations that ganged up against her in 2 Chronicles 20.

Sometimes a physical manifestation doesn't appear. A spouse still walked out, or the child still died from that disease. Yet in every case each moment spent in fasting and prayer results in God-moments and in life-renewing, God-shaping opportunities. As the Bible promises, "The effective, fervent prayer of a righteous man accomplishes much" (James 5:16, MEV). Given these words, we should make engaging the God of glory in intense, belief-filled, petition-making prayers a way of life.

Hezekiah is an outstanding example of someone suffering from a fatal illness and successfully praying for its reversal. The story appears in 2 Kings 20:1–11, when word came to him to prepare his household since he would not recover. The message of his imminent death was more devastating because it came from a prophet, Isaiah. In Israel people consulted the prophet because he heard from God, and God heard his prayers and petitions. However, what Hezekiah expected would be a source of hope instead became bad news. In the same vein when a knowledgeable and dedicated doctor brings us bad news, it does seem that all hope is lost.

But in this case, rather than give in to despair, Hezekiah turned to God in prayer. He poured out his soul. He cried, pleaded, and worshipped. No meaningless, vain repetition of empty words here. Hezekiah spoke to God straight from the heart. He didn't use King James English or pious phrases. His life was at stake; only God could help him. In this case the answer came immediately. Before the prophet had gone far, God spoke to him again. Now, He delivers good news: go and tell Hezekiah he will live another fifteen years. And sure enough, the king recovered and lived.

We won't always experience such quick, dramatic reversals in our situations. Still, I think the story of Hezekiah encourages us to try—to engage God wholeheartedly and make specific petitions to Him in times of life's crises. He will always answer. These answers may manifest themselves in different forms, but they certainly will manifest. Take the opportunity fasting offers to pray fervent, heartfelt, deep-from-the-soul intercession to God. You may be surprised at what you hear and learn.

Dealing with ordinary life

There are different kinds of troubles or hardships that confront us periodically in life's journey. They don't have to be death-dealing hardships like Hezekiah encountered. Instead, they can be problems related to ordinary, everyday life. Situations such as child-care problems (which may not sound too stressful unless you're the parent trying to resolve them), being misunderstood and misrepresented at work, or being betrayed by a close friend. Whatever it is, James delivers one prescription: pray.

Modern culture often caricatures prayer as a form of weakness. Those of us who live in more advanced economies often can find alternatives. Even Christians are guilty of consistently explaining away the need for engaging, expectant prayer. We know the doctor will take care of our ailments, the insurance company will compensate us against unexpected loss, or the courts will administer justice on our behalf. So although we claim to believe in prayer, if many of us are honest, we will admit that our prayers are often perfunctory, glib, and non-expectant. Even when heartfelt, they are only one of many options.

Yet, for the brother of Jesus, there is only one thing we must do when facing trouble or difficulty. Yes, we may need to do other things to follow up, but James is insistent on the need to pray. He knows the power of prayer. In the fifth chapter of his book he recommends prayer for anyone who is suffering or sick, since the prayer of faith will save the sick, raise him up, and bring forgiveness of sins. Earnest prayer from a believing, trusting Christian produces wonderful results. *Your* prayer "has great power and produces wonderful results" (James 5:16, NLT). Do you believe that? If so, you will *take* the time to pray regarding that hardship, disappointment, or problem at work. Incorporate earnest, believing prayer into your fasting periods and trust God to produce wonderful results, in His own way and His own time.

Prayers of praise

Prayers during fasting don't have to only concern desperate situations. Life is not just about troubles. It is often filled with such blessings as a new baby, a new job, a joyous family vacation, and friendships. Life is good. James asks the question (and answers it): "Are any of you happy? You should sing praises" (James 5:13, NLT).

Most days will be pleasant. So, when we are feeling blessed, cheerful, and joyful, we should let God know about it by singing praises, hymns, and psalms, and thanking Him for His provision. Indeed, fasting tends to be even more rewarding when we incorporate a component of awe and wonder in God's presence. When we stay long enough and committed enough in His presence while fasting and praying, we are much more likely to catch a glimpse of His glory and a ray of His ineffable light. Dazzled by His person, we exclaim with joy—as did the psalmist—such phrases as:

- "How excellent is Your name in all the earth!" (Ps. 8:1, MEV).

- "The earth is full of the goodness of the LORD" (Ps. 33:5, NKJV).

- "If it had not been the LORD who was on our side, when men rose up against us, then they would have swallowed us alive" (Ps. 124:2–3, NKJV).

- "What is man that You are mindful of him, and the son of man that You attend to him?" (Ps. 8:4, MEV).

The psalmist offers us a good example to follow by giving voice to gratitude. Fasting is an excellent time to delve deep into the divine heart by adoring God and admiring Him. When we take the time to extricate ourselves from worldly distractions, we allow ourselves to become present to God. We look into His face and observe His loveliness, His grandeur, and the wonders of His grace. We may open our mouths to tell Him what He means to us, and find that words fail us. In such times we can compensate by singing hymns and making melody in our hearts. We hum under our breath as we marvel how He loves us so.

I invite you to sing this song (psalm) below with David. Read it aloud, or meditate on the words. But either way, let David's effusive praise and wonder reach your own soul as you sing along with him:

> I lift you high in praise, my God, O my King!
>> and I'll bless your name into eternity.
>
> I'll bless you every day,
>> and keep it up from now to eternity.
>
> GOD is magnificent; he can never be praised
>> enough.
>> There are no boundaries to his greatness.
>
> Generation after generation stands in awe of your
>> work;
>> each one tells stories of your mighty acts.
>
> Your beauty and splendor have everyone talking;
>> I compose songs on your wonders.
>
> Your marvelous doings are headline news;
>> I could write a book full of the details of your
>> greatness.
>
> The fame of your goodness spreads across the
>> country;
>> your righteousness is on everyone's lips.
>
> GOD is all mercy and grace—
>> not quick to anger, is rich in love.
>
> GOD is good to one and all;
>> everything he does is suffused with grace.
>
> Creation and creatures applaud you, GOD;
>> your holy people bless you.

They talk about the glories of your rule,
  they exclaim over your splendor,

Letting the world know of your power for good,
  the lavish splendor of your kingdom.

Your kingdom is a kingdom eternal;
  you never get voted out of office.

GOD always does what he says,
  and is gracious in everything he does.

GOD gives a hand to those down on their luck,
  gives a fresh start to those ready to quit.

All eyes are on you, expectant;
  you give them their meals on time.

Generous to a fault,
  you lavish your favor on all creatures.

Everything GOD does is right—
  the trademark on all his works is love.

GOD's there, listening for all who pray,
  for all who pray and mean it.

He does what's best for those who fear him—
  hears them call out, and saves them.

GOD sticks by all who love him,
  but it's all over for those who don't.

My mouth is filled with GOD's praise.
  Let everything living bless him,
  bless his holy name from now to eternity.
                    —PSALM 145:1–21

Chapter 15

DIVINE GUIDANCE

So watch your step. Use your head. Make the most of every chance you get. These are desperate times! Don't live carelessly, unthinkingly. Make sure you understand what the Master wants.

—Ephesians 5:16–17

David inquired of the Lord, "Shall I pursue this raiding party? Will I overtake them?" "Pursue them," he answered. "You will certainly overtake them and succeed in the rescue."

—1 Samuel 30:8, niv

T HE CONSECRATION AND PRAYERFUL MODE PROVIDED by fasting is a good opportunity to seek divine guidance. From personal to corporate matters God wants to share His wisdom with us. Each new day in this land of the living is like arriving in a new territory. Each day brings fresh opportunities—and fresh trials. We never quite know which step will bring us to a turn in which blessings await us, or when a fresh misunderstanding or pain may be lurking. To survive and thrive, you have to watch your step, use your head, and make the most of every opportunity.

But this watchfulness is not a result of fear of being swallowed up by the "giants" in the land that struck fear in the hearts of most of the Israeli spies (Num. 13–14), it is born out of a desire to understand what the Lord wants. We shouldn't live in this territory of faith shriveled up in fear and debilitating passions of worry and anxiety, walking about ever cautious and timid. Instead, we can live freely and fully—as we understand God's will. Understanding the will of the Lord frees us to *pursue* life in that direction, freely and joyfully maximizing every opportunity.

As author Eugene Peterson puts in his popular paraphrase of Scripture that I quoted at the start of this chapter: "Make sure you understand what the Master wants." Do you know what God wants in your current situation? To be sure, this doesn't mean being rock-solid certain about everything that is going to happen to you, or a certainty regarding that grand plan God has for you for the next fifty years. This kind of knowing what God wants means taking each step prayerfully and listening for His guidance.

We live in an age that believes that we basically know almost everything there is to know. We live in a drive-through culture that features drive-through pharmacies, drive-through restaurants, drive-through grocery stores, and drive-through gas stations—even drive-through medical clinics. Given the convenience-oriented culture in which Westerners live, we can fall prey to the idea that God should communicate His divine guidance in the same method while we drive through life's busy terrain.

Too many people lack the patience and training to seek God's wisdom and guidance through prayer and fasting.

Some may even mock the idea of withdrawing from this busy life for the sole purpose of praying and seeking God's face. Yet there comes a time in every person's walk when life places a demand on them to make crucial, sometimes life-altering decisions. At such times we need the input of friends, pastors, professionals, or loved ones—input often shaped by the limited wisdom of this world. Our human advisors mean well and may be very knowledgeable, but they cannot tell us what tomorrow brings.

Only God knows the future. He knows where we are headed, the path we will follow, and our final destination. He knows the hearts of the people with whom we deal. He even knows our hearts better than we do. Sometimes we lie to ourselves so much that we begin to believe those lies. God knows the true condition of our hearts, and still loves us. He is committed to us because of His immense love. He is truth. In times of decisions, big or small, He wants us to consult with Him. In those life-defining decisions, we need to consult Him. Times of fasting are wonderful opportunities to ask for God's direction and guidance on specific issues.

Waiting on God

The leaders of the church at Antioch took God's guidance seriously in their work as ministers. All gathered to fast and pray for God's guidance to lead the people and serve as God wanted them to serve. They expected God to lead them: "One day as they were worshiping God—they were also fasting as they waited for guidance—the Holy

Spirit spoke: 'Take Barnabas and Saul and commission them for the work I have called them to do'" (Acts 13:2).

The act of fasting as these early church fathers waited for guidance is highly significant.

I get a mental picture of a group of leaders who gave up all other important assignments, just to wait for God's guidance. They prayed, sang songs, and listened. All the while, they fasted.

I wonder what will happen if this kind of image is duplicated among church leaders in congregations across the United States. Imagine the pastor and church leaders fasting and waiting on God—not to endorse a decision the pastor has already made, or to provide money to fund the next building project, but to hear what the Lord has to say. Not that there is anything wrong with making quick decisions (God gave us a capable mind for that reason) or carrying out a new project. But what if the Lord directed those decisions? Or gave His specific word regarding those projects?

Those leaders from Antioch were prophets and teachers. They could hear from God, and they knew the Scriptures inside and out. And still they waited and fasted until they heard from the Lord, corporately. I don't know about you, but I find something incredibly moving about that picture. After all, any one of those men could have presumptuously claimed to know God's will, either because of title, position, or past accomplishments. But none of them did. Instead, together, as brothers in Christ, they fasted, prayed, and sought God's guidance until He spoke.

When God spoke, He asked them to release Paul and Barnabas unto the work He had called them to do. So, in obedience, these leaders blessed Paul and Barnabas and sent them out. Today Christendom is the better for it, since Paul and Barnabas went on to reach many unreached peoples. Later, Paul wrote the epistles that continue to be a blessing to Christians of all generations. Yet I ask: What if these leaders had not been attentive to the will of the Lord? What if they did not understand His will? Or what if they insisted that these two talented men might as well serve out whatever calling they had in the local church at Antioch—loyal, submissive, and supportive of their pastor while they waited for their "time"? Would we still have had the kind of Paul who emerged? What if they had felt threatened by Paul's revelation from Christ and tried to put him under?

We don't know what would have happened if those men had not responded to the will of the Lord, but today we are glad that they did. Fasting and worshipful prayer helped them discern God's will. While seeking God's guidance, they realized now was the time to let go of these two men to serve God as He had called them—not grudgingly, but joyfully.

David seeks God

If the church leaders at Antioch provided a good example of seeking guidance from God as a group, David provides an example of an individual intent on celebrating God's guidance at every turn. David was not a perfect man by any standard. Still, one of the things that ultimately made David successful was his choice to constantly seek God's guidance throughout his life.

In one of those seasons David was in transition. You have likely experienced the same kind of "in-between" moments, when you have started on a journey but not quite reached your destination. Life is filled with such transitions. David was there, already ordained to be king of Israel, yet fleeing from his predecessor, Saul, who felt threatened by the young warrior. An anointed king forced to live as a fugitive. Blessed with a great future, but currently living in trials and difficulty. Destined for the palace, but making the desert his home. David's wanderings had finally brought him to Ziklag, where he settled down a bit.

A group of men had followed him around faithfully. They believed in him. As they settled down, this group started families. While David was away, trying to help the president of the region in which he and his supporters were settling, some Amalekites raided his city and took away all their families and belongings, including David's wives. When David returned with his men and saw what had happened, brokenness swept over them. The men who had bonded with David through all the years of pain and trials had suddenly *had enough*. They whispered to each other about stoning David to death.

In the midst of this crisis David did something that is as important as it is revealing about his character. He went in to seek the Lord's face. He wanted to get a word from God about what he should do: Should he pursue the raiders? Would he be able to recover their family members alive? Or would pursuing these Amalekites only embolden them to kill their wives and children? Was it better to leave them as servants to those infidel Amalekites rather than risk getting them all killed? In the same way as the leaders of the church at Antioch David waited for God to speak. Finally God spoke: "Pursue them. You will certainly overtake them and succeed in the rescue" (1 Sam. 30:8, NIV).

Now, since David knows God's will, in pursuing after the raiders he would not be acting recklessly or thoughtlessly. He would succeed in rescuing his supporters' families and their possessions. Oh the joy of understanding the will of the Lord and receiving His clear guidance! Now, David knew the assurance of God's encouragement. When he spoke, his followers knew there was hope too. They quickly dropped the thought of killing David and marched with him as they pursued the band of raiders. And yes, they recovered all their family members and their belongings, as well as extra bounty.

God's guidance helps us recover the fullness of life. It helps us recover hope and joy in believing. God's direction helps us avoid needless heartaches. And fasting provides the intensity and focus to seek God and wait until we hear His voice. We wait and wait, no matter how long it takes. We listen, intently and expectantly, until He offers His guidance.

Here is the thing that never ceases to amaze me: whenever we eagerly seek Him, in His mercy God tends to reveal His will. He spoke to the leadership at Antioch. He spoke to David. Through Eli the prophet He spoke to Hannah as she prayed (1 Sam. 2). Each of these examples demonstrates how God longs to guide us and direct our paths, no matter what our church background. When you fast, ask Him specifically to lead you to make the right decisions. Life is a series of choices and decisions; one bad choice often leads to another. However, when we engage God through prayer and fasting, we surrender long enough to hear His direction.

Making time for God

How do I receive guidance from the Lord? It may sound simplistic, but it is a matter of making time to be alone with God. This is where fasting may be helpful. You dedicate a time frame to be alone, where you can confess your sins and pride to the Lord. Often a prideful heart is difficult to lead. Discuss whatever issue concerns you with the Lord as you would with a close friend. I often keep a piece of paper on which I write down the pros and cons, or the reasons for or against, a particular decision or idea. I directly ask the Lord for His wisdom and guidance.

Like the leaders at Antioch, each of us is to pray but also worship. We give God glory. We bless and extol His name as we revel in His wonders and gaze into His face. We study the Scriptures and let His Word speak to us privately. This allows Him to reveal hidden motives or arrogance or false assumptions we are harboring. We may get up from our knees without a clear word, but we are sure that, somehow, He will lead the way. This helps us to step out with more confidence, assured that He will guide us.

The only easy-to-follow guide to hearing from the Lord is to give ourselves completely to Him, then listen and obey. In that regard, I like how *The Message Bible* puts it: "So here's what I want you to do, God helping you: Take your everyday, ordinary life—your sleeping, eating, going-to-work, and walking-around life—and place it before God as an offering. Embracing what God does for you is the best thing you can do for him. Don't become so well-adjusted to your culture that you fit into it without even thinking. Instead, fix your attention on God. You'll be changed from the inside out. Readily recognize what he wants from you, and quickly respond to it. Unlike the culture around you, always dragging you down to its level of immaturity, God brings the best out of you, develops well-formed maturity in you" (Rom. 12:1–2).

The very first step to being readily led by God is a decision to take our everyday, ordinary lives and place them before God as an offering. Our waking, our going to school, our marriage, our work, nursing a baby—whatever the task, dedicate it to Him. Giving every aspect of life to God marks the start of receiving divine guidance. Letting God into the "daily-ness" of our journey is a pleasing offering. Why? Because He loves us so much He wants to be a part of our daily lives. He wants to participate and take an active lead in them. When God becomes the center around which we carry out the routines of life, it is much easier for us to receive His guidance during life-defining moments.

As Peterson renders it: "Embracing what God does for you is the best thing you can do for him." Understanding and following the will of the Lord involves embracing what God is doing for you and in you—right now, in this very place. What is God doing? Not what do we want to do, but what is God working out for us and through us? We may become so adjusted to our own way of doing things that we are not really paying attention to what God is doing. We may become so consumed by what culture says is the right way that we do not pay attention to God's way. We may become so consumed in our "rightness" that we stop listening for God's wisdom.

Understanding the will of the Lord requires paying attention to God and to His works and His ways. He is working in us so that we both desire His will and do it. When we look up and away from our wants and desires, we may be fortunate enough to recognize what He wants from us. Sometimes we fight with the idea of where we are located, or the people we are associated with, so much that we don't recognize what God is doing or saying through them. During fasting, as I discussed earlier, we wait on God long enough to see clearly what God is doing and fully embrace it. Saying yes to God is the beginning of finding the freedom to follow in His steps. Fasting, with the conditions of humility and surrender that it engenders, fosters listening and responding to God's will.

Chapter 16

PRAYING THE SCRIPTURES

God is our Refuge and Strength [mighty and impenetrable to
temptation], a very present and well-proved help in trouble.

—Psalm 46:1, AMP

The abstinence is not to be an end in itself but rather for the purpose of being separated to the Lord and to concentrate on godliness. This kind of fasting reduces the influence of our own self-will
and invites the Holy Spirit to do a more intense work in us.

—Bible professor Bill Thrasher[1]

HERE IS SOMETHING TRULY RESTORATIVE AND
formative in engaging the Holy Scriptures during prayer
and fasting. God's salvation is embedded in these words
of life. They earned that label for a reason: God's life saturates
them. As we meditate on His words, God's life becomes light,
shining brightly across the darkness of this world and life's
temptations, trials, and pains. When we search the Scriptures, we should engage them with all our hearts, because

within them is the essence of life. God's Word contains His power to save, restore, bless, encourage, correct, and refresh. Fasting becomes more profitable when we devote time to ingesting His holy words. We sing His words, read them, and pray them. The words of Scripture even have a way of expressing clearly what our spirits are feeling.

For example, take the psalms. I am continually amazed at the depth of humanity revealed in their words, whether struggles, sins, triumphs, enemy problems, jealousy issues, or the betrayal of close friends. I am even more amazed at the ability of the psalmist to express my soul's deepest prayers. Sometimes as I meditate on them, my soul cries, "Yes!" I am drawn to a place where I receive the right words to pray out the longing and groaning of my innermost being. It seems as if there is always a scripture or psalm that suits every moment, whether times of intense joy or desperate pain.

Allow me to share how I engage the psalms in prayer. (Of course, everyone tends to approach Scripture differently, so there is no prescription about how you ought to allow scriptures to instruct and guide you.) I start by meditating quietly on Scripture and allowing it to speak to me, search my heart, and heal any evil way in me. Then I pray with these scriptures. I often will use a psalm as a tool to allow the Holy Spirit to pray through me and for me. You may ask, "What does praying the Scriptures look like?" I don't know what that looks like for others, but for me it involves taking up each verse, praying the words out loud, rephrasing the words to suit the cry or pain in my heart, and turning those words of Scripture to words of prayer toward God.

Praying Psalm 46

Here is what praying the Scriptures might look like if I were praying with Psalm 46, using the New International Version. Since this is meant as a personal prayer, I use a lot of expressions of "me," "I," and "mine." Still, I hope you will take my words to mean you personally. Pray and say those words back to God, because, in the words of the late Carl Rogers, noted psychologist, "What is most personal is most universal."[2]

God is our refuge and strength, an ever-present help in trouble (v. 1).

> *God, thank You for being my refuge and strength. You have been a refuge, a shelter, and a place of protection for believers in ages past. You are my present refuge. I run to You, O Lord, for protection from the troubles I am in right now. My mind may be in turmoil about this circumstance, but I come into Your shelter. Bring me peace from the storm. Lord, You are a storm shelter for me and my family from the adverse winds of life. Lord, You are also my strength, my anchor, and my stay. I receive Your strength for today. God, You are a very present help for me in time of trouble. I come to You, knowing that You are present, strong, and willing to help me. You are a present help. I know I needed Your help yesterday, but You are still my present help today in any trouble. You are the help I need. So, I have come to You, dear Lord. Here I am before my refuge and strength. The God of heaven is my*

refuge. *The God of heaven is my strength. The God of angel armies is an ever-present help for me. I rejoice in You, rock of my salvation.*

Therefore we will not fear, though the earth give way and the mountains fall into the heart of the sea, though its waters roar and foam and the mountains quake with their surging (vv. 2–3).

O God, because You are my refuge and strength and an ever-present help in trouble, I choose not to fear. In the name of Jesus Christ, I reject fear and agitating passions. I receive freedom from worry and anxiety. I know that physically the waters of life seem to be roaring against me right now, but I choose to be calm in Your presence. I receive Your peace, because You will give them perfect peace whose mind is stayed on You. I stay my mind on You, my refuge and strength. The mountain of obstacles seems to be mounting, but in the name of Jesus, I choose to rejoice in God, my Maker. You are my stay and anchor. As the mountains surround Jerusalem, so Your strength and shelter surround me. I am hid in Christ and Christ in God. My life is hid in You, O God, my refuge and strength. I uproot fear from my mind. I cast down imaginations that sow seeds of fear and anxiety in my mind. I trust in You to shelter my mind, even in this turmoil.

There is a river whose streams make glad the city of God, the holy place where the Most High dwells (v. 4).

God, You have left us a river, the Holy Spirit, whose streams make glad the city of God, the church of the living God. Your Holy Spirit lives and moves in the congregation of believers, and He also lives and moves in my heart. Oh, may Your streams make glad my heart. Make glad my home. Make glad my children. I present myself and mine as a holy place for Your dwelling. Did Jesus not say that for those who believe, out of their innermost being will flow rivers of living waters? According to Your Word, by this He meant the Holy Spirit whom those who believe will receive. Thank You, Lord, that You have given me the Holy Spirit. I pray now that His rivers of living, refreshing water will flow out of my innermost belly. May the joy and renewal that come from the Holy Spirit emanate from my innermost being right now.

God is within her, she will not fall; God will help her at break of day (v. 5).

Hallelujah! God is within me. I will not fall. I will not fail. God will help me, and early. A new day is coming—the dawn of His help. I will stay fixed in His will; He will help me right on time. I am going to keep following the right path, because He will help me at the break of dawn. Weeping may last for a night, but His joy comes in the morning. Morning will come. This night season will be over eventually. His strength will keep me through the night. God, who is within me, the God of our Lord Jesus Christ, will help me.

Nations are in uproar, kingdoms fall; he lifts his voice, the earth melts. The LORD Almighty is with us; the God of Jacob is our fortress (vv. 6–7).

Yes, I know that the economy is bad. I know that those big corporations are laying off employees. I know that there are economic, political, and biological forces at play that cannot just be ignored or wished away. But the Lord Almighty is with me. The God of Jacob, the God who helped even cheating, conniving Jacob, is with me. He has chosen to be my fortress, my refuge. It is not by works, lest anyone should boast. It is by grace that we are saved. His grace alone is my redemption. His shelter is strong enough to withstand every wind of economic, political, or biological change. The God of Jacob is my fortress!

Come and see what the LORD has done, the desolations he has brought on the earth. He makes wars cease to the ends of the earth. He breaks the bow and shatters the spear; he burns the shields with fire (vv. 8–9).

Oh, enemy of my soul, come and see what the Lord does. You thought you had thrown a death-dealing curveball at me, but God makes wars to cease. God breaks the bows and shatters the spear of war. God has taken what you meant for evil and has turned it around for my good. God is turning my mourning into joy. He is giving me the oil of joy for any heaviness. God is taking my mistakes and using them for His glory. God is turning those kids hooked on drugs around and using them for His glory. Oh, come and see what God can do with a life given over to Him. I give You my life, God. Take it up and make the wars cease. Break the bows, spears, and weapons of war fashioned against me. Bring me to a place of refreshing grace. Renew my life again.

He says, "Be still, and know that I am God; I will be exalted among the nations, I will be exalted in the earth" (v. 10).

God has said to me: "Be still and know that I am God." Now, my soul says yes to God. Dear Lord, I choose to be still, to stop fretting, and to yield all to You. I know You are going to show Yourself as God, the Almighty One. You will be exalted in my life and circumstances. Your glory will be revealed in my world. Be exalted in my decisions, my daily walk, and my actions. Teach me to be still. Teach me to let You fight battles in my life. Help me to stop struggling and constantly fighting. I choose to let You take control, to defend me and advocate for me. I will be still and know that You are God.

The LORD Almighty is with us; the God of Jacob is our fortress (v. 11).

> *That is my hope and confidence: that the One who is sovereign and reigns supreme is for me. You are on my side. The God who patiently worked in Jacob until he became the Israel of God is with me. He is on my side. You are not giving up on me. You are still working in me. You have a plan to make me the person you want me to become. My heart rejoices in the fact that the God of Jacob is my fortress through life. I breathe easy. I rest secure in Your love. Thank You for being my refuge and strength. Amen.*

Chapter 17

FASTING AND FORGIVENESS

This is the kind of fast day I'm after: to break the chains of injustice, get rid of exploitation in the workplace, free the oppressed, cancel debts.

—ISAIAH 58:6

Fasting is the soul of prayer; mercy is the lifeblood of fasting....So, if you pray, fast; if you fast, show mercy; if you want your petition to be heard, hear the petition of others. If you do not close your ear to others, you open God's ear to yourself.

**—SAINT PETER CHRYSOLOGUS (1380–1450)
KNOWN AS THE "DOCTOR OF HOMILIES"[1]**

WHILE DOING RESEARCH FOR THE FIRST PART of this book, it stunned me to learn that according to the CDC, the rates of depression and divorce appear to be higher in socially conservative and evangelical Protestant areas; namely, such states as Arkansas, Alabama, Mississippi, Louisiana, Tennessee, and Oklahoma.[2] I found it astonishing that in states where Christian values and culture supposedly predominate, people could be in such a sad condition. Christ is the Prince of Peace, so peace should be a visible part of our walk with Him. And as studies indicate, poverty and higher overall marriage rates do not fully account for this curious fact.[3]

While social scientists continue to research this and find convincing explanations, one thing is clear to me: such statistics pose a wake-up call to Christians. We must examine how our professed doctrines square with the reality of our day-to-day lives. Such social realities should drive us to our knees as we humble ourselves before God—and admit that we too are affected by this broken world. We don't have it all together. We struggle just like the rest of the world and endure some of the same heartaches. Life-leaking events happen to us all. Still, I wonder whether more real-life practicing of forgiveness might help to heal our hearts and millions of broken relationships.

Damaging moments need not be fatal to relationships; our hurts and brokenness can be healed. This reality is the only hope for weary travelers to find healing and restorative moments beside the "still waters" the psalmist refers to in Psalm 23:2. Fasting can provide such moments in which God can tend to our wounds, console our hurting hearts, bind up our broken spirits, and relieve our grieving souls of bitterness and sorrow. While many fail to see spiritual fasting as an opportunity for life-restoring moments, that is precisely its purpose. It offers moments to retract ourselves from everyday distractions in order to wait on God and find refreshing in His presence. It is a time to allow the divine hand of grace to reach deep down into our hurting souls and bring lasting healing. This can involve numerous personal offenses, hurts, letdowns, and harsh words that have accumulated over many years.

Fasting is a time when we stay quiet in God's presence long enough to allow Him to clean up the wellsprings of daily life. Wise Solomon advised: "Keep vigilant watch over your heart; that's where life starts" (Prov. 4:23). The heart is indeed the wellspring of life. If it becomes muddled with bitterness, anxiety, or despair, then the life that issues from it becomes equally muddled. In fasting we present our hearts—whether angry, joyous, or indifferent—before the God who sees all and knows all.

Key to healing

Fasting provides healing opportunities, but it does not offer healing by itself. We must accept the healing that is offered by the Holy Spirit. In fasting, as we lie beside the "still waters" of grace, we place our hearts in these healing waters. We pray and ask for God's healing, mercy, and kindness. However, we must also offer that same grace to others. We forgive as God has forgiven us. When we couple fasting with forgiveness, healing forces flow over us. Fasting is a moment to focus on what is important in life, such as family, our spouse, friends, goodwill, love, and goodness. When that focus comes into view, we reflect and ponder on God's light-dazzling glory. We can see more clearly in the light of His extravagant grace. We view the injuries and injustices of life through the vast prism of His kindness and eternity.

Such a divine view will enable us to be more apt to give the benefit of the doubt to others and, where necessary, to forgive. Fasting provides the time and focus, and prayer provides the divine connection, but we must still act to wash our hearts in the streams of God's forgiving grace. We have to say yes to more than God's forgiveness. We must choose to extend that forgiveness to others on life's journey. Fasting periods offer powerful moments to forgive and be forgiven.

As the prophet Isaiah observed, true fasting includes freeing the oppressed and canceling debts, whether personal, financial, or emotional. Fasting cancels debts. Given the sad state of marriage and personal relationships in so many places where people espouse a belief in Jesus, I must raise the question: Could forgiveness—this canceling of debts—help curb issues such as high divorce rates? Is it possible that most divorces stem from an accumulation of unforgiven, unresolved pain and resentment?

Life is relational, personal, and local. The more intimate a relationship, the greater the tendency to allow pain and resentment to build up. When we feel offended or taken for granted, we may say something about it, but ultimately silently stick it on our "offense shelf" with many others. Whether we sort them by date, severity, or other criteria, we still store them up.

"They should know better," we tell ourselves. Yet we hold back because it hurts too deeply to engage our spouses. "How could he, after all that I've done for him?" "How could she treat me like that—with no respect?" As legendary poet William Blake observed, "It is easier to forgive an enemy than to forgive a friend."4 The wounds from a friend are more painful, because we have given something of ourselves in the process. Our hearts are involved, and our expectations are high. We hope for the best and endeavor in spite of ourselves to give the best.

What can be more personal and more intimate than the marriage relationship? In marriage we forsake all others and commit to this one person. We share all—spirit, soul, and body. We open up ourselves. When this significant other hurts us, it hurts deeply. At first we may tell ourselves that he or she "meant well." So we give our spouses the benefit of the doubt. But then, after a while, we become "wiser." Close friends may tell us that we are being played for a fool by letting go and moving on. The real danger comes when the enemy of our soul questions the intentions of our loved ones. Pretty soon we will take Satan's cue and do the same. Offenses that would have been easily overlooked or readily forgiven in the past are now filed away as unresolved. We smile and carry on as though everything is OK.

Even if we express discontent, we do so in such a cautious way that our spouses assume it's no big deal. Yet we are muddying the waters in our hearts with resentment and a desire for revenge. It builds up until one day we wake up determined to deal with it *once and for all.* Such is the story of many a divorce, as well as other broken family relationships or friendships.

Maximum forgiveness

In Isaiah 58 I see the prophet saying that instead of waiting to serve a divorce paper or get even with another person who has wronged us, we can use a period of fasting to cancel this debt. Forgiveness is never easy, especially when it involves such things as a spouse's slights or betrayal by a close friend. Yet fasting can help with this challenging process. As we wait on God and refocus on His marvelous grace, we stay still enough—for long enough—in the Potter's house that He can free us of pain and resentment.

We don't gloss over the offense or pretend it is not there. We should always be honest and open with God. But when we surrender our hearts, we ask for His fresh touch. Then we wait patiently for His answers. Fasting and prayer are never a quick fix; serious fasting is personal, deeply honest, and painstakingly deliberate. After we surrender, we wait, maybe shed some tears, and keep praying as we seek to lay down our burdens. The fasting that God approves of is the fast that releases the oppressed and cancels the debt. We give up our need for revenge or desire to see misfortune fall on the object of our anger. Once God frees us from the oppression of unforgiveness and vengeful thoughts, we are free to forgive others and cancel their debts—even if they haven't asked for forgiveness.

Peter got a practical lesson from Jesus on this "believing and forgiving" lifestyle the day he asked the Savior, "'Lord, how often shall my brother sin against me, and I forgive him? Up to seven times?'" (Matt. 18:21, NKJV). The Bible doesn't indicate whether Peter spoke from personal experience. For the sake of this discussion, let's assume he did. If so, it would appear that Peter had been enduring and letting go of an offense from this brother or sister. He may have forgiven six times; now he had to forgive *a seventh*? I can hear the thought rolling around Peter's mind: "Seven times; that has to be the limit." How could anyone reasonably expect him to forgive the same person more than seven times without exacting some revenge? After all, Peter was only human. He must have expected Jesus to validate him. Surely forgiving the same person seven times deserved a celebration. Surely even Jesus would understand if Peter reacted angrily and vengefully against this brother or sister after seven instances of extending grace.

Jesus surprised Peter with His straightforward advice: "'I do not say to you, up to seven times, but up to seventy times seven'" (Matt. 18:22, NKJV). To accumulate 490 offenses from one person has to take two things. First, that person has to spend a significant portion of their time with you (think about a spouse, a child, a parent, or a close friend). Second, it will take a lifetime of accumulating offenses. That can be devastating—if we don't stop long enough in God's presence to give it all up and shed the grip of bitterness and resentment. Fasting provides a time of consecration, which allows God to reach down and uproot bitterness from our lives.

Forgiveness in action

Before Peter could get self-righteous or indignant over what Jesus was asking, or before he could protest ("Lord, this is incredibly difficult; do You know how tough that would be?"), Jesus offers a powerful parable about forgiveness. It concerned a wealthy king who was owed the equivalent of several million dollars by one of his servants, a man I'll call Jerry. When the master demanded repayment, the servant begged for more time. He asked the master to be patient; he intended to pay up despite the enormity of his debt. For some reason the master had compassion on him and decided to forgive this enormous debt. Naturally

Jerry responded with joy. He knew that he didn't deserve this kind of huge favor. Truth be told, he couldn't pay the debt even with a lifetime of his earnings.

Jerry must have told all the other servants, because everyone knew about his good fortune. However, the next day while going about his business—glad to be alive, and thankful for the break life had delivered—the man encountered another servant whom I will call Tom. He owed Jerry a relative pittance (some biblical scholars say less than twenty dollars). Tom likely stopped to congratulate Jerry and rejoice with him. After the banter that followed, Jerry asked about Tom's debt to him. Tom felt bad about his inability to pay but promised to do so soon. He asked Jerry for patience and understanding as he worked to repay his loan. "Surely he understands," Tom thought. "After all, he has just been forgiven a much bigger debt by our master."

To his surprise, the ungrateful Jerry brought the full wrath of the law to bear on Tom. He took Tom to court, and when he couldn't pay the debt, Jerry demanded that Tom be imprisoned until he could.

Of course, the next working day Tom didn't show up for work. Another servant made some inquiries and discovered Tom was in prison, on account of the debt owed to his fellow servant. Furious, the other servants reported these events to the king, who couldn't believe it. "Jerry did what? After I forgave him millions of dollars in debt?" The master rescinded the debt forgiveness he had offered and threw Jerry in jail until he could repay his multimillion-dollar debt. The obvious conclusion:

Jerry will never get out. (You can read the whole story in Matthew 18:21–35.)

You can likely guess the moral of this story: in light of the huge debt of sin and depravity from which God forgave us, the offenses we have endured from our spouses, family, friends, neighbors, and coworkers pale in comparison. God knows we will get hurt in life, sometimes in measures that are exceedingly unjust. And He still expects us to forgive. No, that doesn't mean they are not devastating, especially when the slights come from loved ones and friends. It doesn't minimize the pain we feel from these offenses. Still, when we focus on His extravagant grace, His touch of kindness should soften us enough that we extend the same forgiveness to others.

Deep wounds

This isn't easy. After all, a wound from a friend hurts deeper than one from an enemy. When we act on a human level and recoil with anger, we may seek to attack in a mode of vengeance, or seethe with silent bitterness and resentment. Yet, what happens if the person who offended us begs for forgiveness? Or asks for time to change and grow? Or in the case of a financial debt asks us to be patient?

Consider that before God, we have asked for and received His patience and kindness. He knows us more than anyone else, and He still loves us. This should encourage us and bring us healing and hope. Despite our mistakes, He lavishes His forgiveness and love on us. God is still working on us, and we know He isn't done with us. We are certainly a work in progress. The divine heart gives us the benefit of the doubt, and repeatedly offers a second chance.

Yet in our pain and frustration with other fallible human beings, we can easily forget that God calls us to extend some of that grace to others. In other words, He asks us to give the benefit of the doubt to that brother, sister, friend, or spouse who constantly gets on our nerves. If we react in anger and unforgiveness, and lose sight of God's mercy, we imprison others in our hearts. Yes, some of their offenses are serious; compared to eternity, though, they are quite frivolous. As the parable in Matthew 18 shows, when we lock people up in our minds, we suffer imprisonment with them. We aren't free to be who we are—how could we, with that burden within our soul?

Releasing the prison door and letting those who hurt us go free is tough to do, especially when they have not asked for our forgiveness. Still, it is the only way to free ourselves from enslavement to the cord of bitterness. Christian theologian and author Lewis Smedes was right when he said, "To forgive is to set a prisoner free and discover that the prisoner was you."[5]

Forgiveness is the only way to free our destiny from destruction. It is the only way to recover the grace of God as we journey through life. Perfunctory prayer won't do it. Just hearing exhortation to forgive on Sunday mornings alone is not enough. Reaching the place of lasting forgiveness does not come except through fasting and prayer. In the place of fasting, we commit to God's presence and His healing touch intensely enough to allow Him to soften our hearts, remove our self-righteousness, and break our all-too-human pride with His love.

It is likely that many have never thought of fasting this way. Too many of us have learned to think of Christian fasting as a time to go and demand things from God— to force His hand, so to speak. But there is exhilarating power awaiting those who intentionally integrate fasting and forgiveness. A good part of the stress we encounter has to do with relationships, whether at home, work, school, or church. It is true that some types of depressive disorders have something to do with neurochemical imbalance. Yet it is also true that stress is an important factor in depression.

Loss of a loved one leaves us numb and unfeeling. News of a major illness leaves us in pain and afraid. If a spouse walks out on us, we feel rejected and abandoned. All are high-stress events that leave us feeling angry, bitter, and "owed." These are no trivial events. And the feelings of pain and disappointment are no small matter either. Not only is life not fair, but also God doesn't seem to be hearing us or "coming through" for us. Granted, there are no simple solutions in times such as those. This life-journey living is complex and sometimes inexplicable. Still, we can make an effort to present ourselves to the One who can heal hearts and renew our strength.

In fasting we make time to wait on God, tell Him how angry or upset we are, and share our deepest thoughts with Him. When that happens, we may forgive even when life is not fair. When we cancel the debts others owe, we free ourselves from inner oppression. This enables us to continue our journey with new grace. An internal miracle takes place through forgiveness, which leads to other, tangible miracles. It will be a wonderful thing to see more men and women separate themselves to intermittent periods of fasting and prayer, committing themselves to ridding their hearts of resentment and bitterness. I pray a new awareness and awakening will come to the Christian community about the true meaning and ramifications of God-ordained fasting, which will culminate in waves of forgiveness—maybe even the next Great Awakening.

Chapter 18

PRAYER WALKS

If thou wouldst preserve a sound body, use fasting and walking;
if a healthful soul, fasting and praying; walking exercises the
body, praying exercises the soul, fasting cleanses both.

—ENGLISH POET FRANCIS QUARLES (1592–1644)[1]

All truly great thoughts are conceived by walking.

—GERMAN PHILOSOPHER AND ATHEIST FRIEDRICH NIETZSCHE[2]

FRIEDRICH NIETZSCHE MAY BE WRONG ABOUT GOD —dead wrong, if you ask me—but he was certainly onto something when he said that great thoughts are conceived through walking. There is something about walking that refreshes, renews, and allows the spirit within to find expression. When we combine prayer and walking with fasting, it can offer unexpected benefits. For some people, fasting that involves waiting on God in prayers indoors—all day—may be less than attractive. Especially those with an active nature who want to be outside to walk in the park, meditate, or pray. What a holistic blessing we enjoy when we walk and pray during fasting.

Such activity renews and refreshes our spirits, souls, and bodies. Many Christians have yet to enjoy this kind of blessing. I know that some with health problems are hard-pressed to walk, and others can cite reasons to avoid it. Yet there are compelling reasons to include walking in our praying and fasting life.

I have always been intrigued by the way Jesus did most of His intense, life-shaping prayers in wide-open fields, on mountainsides, or in a garden. I believe that was for a good reason. There is something about being out in nature that draws us closer to God. It helps displace distractions and our often mind-numbing busyness. Out in the woods or other outdoors settings we can slow down, reflect, grow introspective, and look at the big picture.

When we pray in nature, our prayers are often more sincere, unforced, heartfelt, and relaxed. If we are already in fasting mode, we are all the more eager to listen to God and His wisdom. Creative thoughts flow more easily. Thoughts of forgiveness flash more readily through our minds as we watch the beauty of a sunset. Thoughts of hope fill our minds as we watch the grandeur of a sunrise. All the while, we are praying, listening, and looking up to the God who is Alpha and Omega. No wonder Jesus often prayed outside, especially when He had an important decision to make.

One of those looming decisions early in Jesus's ministry was choosing twelve close followers to whom He would commit the responsibility of continuing His mission on Earth. He had to choose just twelve out of thousands of followers. If He chose wrongly, God's plan might be jeopardized. If they were all saints, then a "Judas" would be missing. Then who would betray Him so as to fulfill His Father's plan? But if He chose more than one Judas, then there might be a big crack in the plan. It had to be eleven saints and only one betrayer. (And who would knowingly choose someone for your inner circle fully aware that they would betray you unto death?)

These were difficult, perplexing choices and decisions. Jesus needed fresh air to clear His head. He needed to be away, alone in nature, so He could pray this through. He could have gone to the temple and shut Himself in, or He could have gone to the house of a close friend. Instead, He took a long walk to the mountainside, and there He prayed. There is nothing doctrinal about this; it is just an observation the gospel writers made about Christ's preference. In fact, He often chose to preach to crowds at a beachside or on a mountaintop.

On this occasion He had a lot on His mind, so He prayed all night. That strikes me as a description of someone who is serious about fasting. He was committed to this time of prayer and was going to stay at it until He had an answer and more clarity about what to do. There is something about taking a walk at the park, on a walking trail, or out in the woods that is both healing and helps us to listen. Jesus walked and prayed. He prayed and walked. He probably stopped, knelt, and prayed. He probably sang songs while out in the open. He probably had some moments of just listening and meditating on the Father. By the time morning came, He had his answer. He knew exactly whom He would choose. He selected His twelve apostles, one of whom was Judas.

Taking a long prayer walk to the mountainside helped Jesus follow His Father's will in making this choice. It seems to me that if praying and walking helped Jesus, it could be beneficial to us too. While we ought to pray at home and at church, we should also consider praying while walking along quiet streets and trails.

Praying in natural settings

In another life-defining moment Jesus needed to have enough time to talk to God about the issue of salvation and His impending death on the cross. After all, this was the primary reason He came to Earth. Now the time was drawing near and the reality of His death coming ever clearer. He knew it was going to be brutal. "Isn't there another way to save the earth without drinking the cup of the shame of the Cross?" Although He knew the mind of the Father, His humanity struggled with the idea. So it was time to pray and settle this with God before it interfered with the Father's divine plan.

With His heart heavy and sorrowful, it was time to engage the Father and settle things in the Spirit: "Then Jesus went with his disciples to a place called Gethsemane, and he said to them, 'Sit here while I go over there and pray'" (Matt. 26:36, NIV). Jesus took three of His closest friends to a garden, of all places. Why not the temple? His choice shows the value of walking outside as He prayed and spoke with God on matters that would affect the world's eternal destiny. Even after that He took a longer walk and prayed. I know that at some point in that walk He stopped, knelt down, and prayed intensely.

After a while He came back to check on His disciples and found them sleeping. He urged them to stay awake and pray. I wonder, if they had been walking, would they have been able to stay awake? Perhaps if they understood the benefits of walking while fasting and praying they may have been more alert. I don't know, but when Jesus came back to check on them after another hour or so, they had fallen asleep again. This time Jesus left them alone. Then He went off again, walking, praying, and pouring His soul out to God. He prayed until He had a breakthrough. He prayed and surrendered all until He could say, freely and joyfully, "Not my will, but yours be done" (Luke 22:42, NIV)! And yet He still knew turmoil. Luke 22:44 says, "And being in anguish, he prayed more earnestly, and his sweat was like drops of blood falling to the ground" (NIV).

I know we are all different people with different inclinations. Still, I believe that everyone can benefit from prayer walks, at least occasionally. Fortunately most cities in this country have parks and recreation centers where people can walk. In every city where my family and I have lived, I have experienced the joy of hours of walking and praying in parks. The mode of my prayer depends on the time of day or the nature of my spiritual need. When the park is busy, I just walk or sit still beside a stream (such as at Island Park in Mount Pleasant, Michigan). Sometimes I head to the park early in the morning or late in the evening, when it is quiet, and pray out my burdens. I walk and pray until I sense a lightening in my spirit or sense God's guidance. When it might be too late for the park, I just walk the streets of our neighborhood.

It doesn't matter what time of year it is either. I like the burst of cold air that fills my lungs in winter, the cool, gentle breezes of spring, the warmth of summer, and the crisp autumn atmosphere. I am especially thankful for a pair of Arkansas attractions: the Crystal Bridges Museum of American Art walking trails in Bentonville and the James Butts Baseball Complex in Siloam Springs. I have walked their trails so often that I thank God for the workers that built them.

Some days my walk is leisurely and meditative. I observe the flowers and walk down to a creek and watch small fish as they swim. I stop to watch kids learning to play baseball or running around the Crystal Bridges trail with their parents scampering after them. On other days I might feel burdened and especially want to take my concerns to the Lord. As I walk, I pray out loud. When overcome by emotion, I let tears fall down my cheeks. Sometimes I veer off into the woods at the Crystal Bridges/Bentonville trails and cry out to God. All the while I inhale the dampness of the air after a fall rain, the scent of budding flowers, or the glory of a sunset. There is something about such scenes that helps clear your head and allows you to listen to God speak to your heart.

The health benefits

I heartily recommend that you consider combining prayer walks and fasting, especially during partial or fruit fasts, when you are more likely to have enough strength. The spiritual and emotional benefits alone are well worth it. For some, it may add additional motivation to know that walking at least thirty minutes a day offers immense benefits in improving several of the conditions discussed earlier in this book. Imagine combining the added benefit of fasting with the benefits of physical activity. According to the American Heart Association, which actively promotes walking, there are eight scientifically documented health benefits of walking.[3]

An example: walking at least thirty minutes a day reduces the risk of coronary heart disease. In fact, in some studies, the risk of heart attack was reduced by about 35 percent in those who walk compared to those who were not engaged in similar activity.[4] Walking has also been shown to improve blood pressure.

Several studies have also shown a correlation between walking and type 2 diabetes prevention rates. A major national clinical trial undertaken to study the impact of weight and physical activity on diabetes, among others, published its results in 2002.[5] Called the Diabetes Prevention Program, the study found that walking only about twenty-one or twenty-two minutes each day (or 150 minutes a week) and losing about 7 percent of one's body weight can reduce the risk of diabetes by 58 percent.[6]

Here is another disease that many people don't know that walking can address: cancer. Walking or other forms of moderate physical activity help reduce the risk of breast cancer and colon cancer. In fact, in one study women who walked briskly for ninety to one hundred twenty minutes each week reduced their risk for breast cancer by 18 percent.[7] Ever experienced the refreshment of a good, long walk? One where your mood improved and you seemed to have a fresh perspective? Well, you are not alone. In one study, people who walked for thirty minutes a day, three to five times a week, reduced the symptoms of depression and enhanced mental well-being by as much as 47 percent.[8]

Other benefits of walking listed on the American Heart Association and Centers for Disease Control and Prevention websites include improved blood lipid profile, reduced risk of osteoporosis, and maintaining a healthy body weight.

Remember, though, that even though physical health is important, your total well-being—spirit, soul, and body—is even more important. When we fast, we reap immense physical and spiritual benefits. When we include prayer in our fasting, we engage with the almighty God. When we include prayer walk in our fasting, we accelerate both the spiritual and physical benefits derived from fasting and prayer.

Remember, too, that you *can* fast. As I mentioned earlier, there are a variety of plans to choose from. I know that some persons have some limitations that affect whether or not they can walk, or how often. However, the majority of persons reading this material can probably walk at least several minutes a day—if you choose to do that. Do it. Walk and pray. Pray and walk as you seek the God of glory. Talk a walk, breathe in fresh air, and let the God of grace give you a new song as you journey through life.

Epilogue

A WORD OF CAUTION

I F YOU ARE SUFFERING FROM A CHRONIC DISEASE SUCH as diabetes, cancer, stroke, or heart problems, you *must* discuss your health with your primary care physician or other specialist before embarking on any kind of fast. You assuredly do not want to follow a protracted fast in hopes of curing yourself of any chronic disease without the supervision of a medical doctor. I have presented fasting not as a disease management program but as a disease prevention practice. I do not recommend fasting for disease management unless your doctor approves and supervises such a plan.

I am not a medical doctor, but a biomedical research scientist. No segment of the foregoing discussion about fasting should be interpreted as any kind of medical prescription. I have done my best to document scientific evidence in support of the health benefits of fasting, as well as a call for a more balanced approach to spiritual fasting. Still, I do not intend to offer any form of medical advice. Fasting is a spiritual discipline that happens to also offer immense health benefits. I highly recommend that you approach fasting from that perspective.

Fasting is beneficial as a lifestyle change for healthy people. It is a disciplined, lifetime habit of reducing your energy intake. The results will be seen through such benefits as the delayed onset of age-associated diseases. As a healthy person, overweight or not, you can benefit—even in small measures—from practicing fasting as defined in this book. However, if you are an individual with major health problems, you are best served by consulting your doctor before initiating any form of fasting.

For all individuals, whether healthy or not, you must consult with your doctor before embarking on any kind of protracted fasting program. In the very least, your doctor will be able to monitor your progress as you fast.

NOTES

CHAPTER 1
WHY FASTING MATTERS

1. "Thomas A. Edison Quotes," GoodReads, accessed September 3, 2015, http://www.goodreads.com/quotes/13639-the-doctor-of-the-future-will-give-no-medication-but.
2. "2014 National Diabetes Statistics Report," Centers for Disease Control and Prevention, October 24, 2014, accessed September 8, 2015, http://www.cdc.gov/diabetes/data/statistics/2014StatisticsReport.html.
3. "Cardiovascular Diseases (CVDs)," World Health Organization, January 2015, accessed September 8, 2015, http://www.who.int/mediacentre/factsheets/fs317/en/.
4. "Cancer Facts & Figures 2015," American Cancer Society, accessed September 8, 2015, http://www.cancer.org/research/cancerfactsstatistics/cancerfactsfigures2015/index.

CHAPTER 2
WHEN LESS IS MORE

1. Mark P. Mattson, "Hormesis Defined," *Ageing Research Reviews* 7, no. 1 (January 2008): 1–7, doi:10.1016/j.arr.2007.08.007.
2. Bronwen Martin, Mark P. Mattson, and Stuart Maudsley, "Caloric Restriction and Intermittent Fasting: Two Potential Diets for Successful Brain Aging," *Ageing Results Reviews* 5, no. 3 (August 2006): 332–353, http://www.ncbi.nlm.nih.gov/pubmed/16899414.
3. Mark P. Mattson, "Dietary Factors, Hormesis and Health," *Ageing Results Reviews* 7, no. 1 (January 2008): 43–48, http://www.ncbi.nlm.nih.gov/pubmed/17913594.
4. Mattson, "Hormesis Defined."
5. Steven A. Schroeder, "We Can Do Better—Improving the Health of the American People," *New England Journal of*

Medicine 357 (September 20, 2007): 1221–1228, accessed September 14, 2015, http://www.nejm.org/doi/full/10.1056/NEJMsa073350.

6.   Ibid.

7.   Ibid.

8.   Ibid.

9.   Ibid.

10.   "Current Cigarette Smoking Among Adults—United States, 2011," Centers for Disease Control and Prevention, *Weekly* 61, no. 44 (November 9, 2012): 889–894, accessed September 8, 2015, http://www.cdc.gov/mmwr/preview/mmwrhtml/mm6144a2.htm.

11.   American Chemical Society, *Chemistry in Context* (New York: McGraw-Hill Higher Education, 2009), 65.

12.   Daniel L. Smith Jr., Tim R. Nagy, and David B. Allison, "Calorie Restriction: What Recent Results Suggest for the Future of Aging Research," *European Journal of Clinical Investigation* 40, no. 5 (May 2010): 440–450, doi:10.1111/j.1365-2362.2010.02276.x.

Chapter 3
Scientifically Speaking

1.   "Fasting Quotes," All About Fasting, accessed September 8, 2015, www.allaboutfasting.com/fasting-quotes.html.

2.   P. Caro et al., "Effect of 40 Percent Restriction of Dietary Amino Acids (Except Methionine) on Mitochondrial Oxidative Stress and Biogenesis, AIF and SIRT1 in Rat Liver," *Biogerontology* 10, no. 5 (October 2009): 579–592, doi:10.1007/s10522-008-9200-4.

3.   Frauke Neff et al., "Rapamycin Extends Murine Lifespan but Has Limited Effects on Aging," *Journal of Clinical Investigation* 123, no. 8 (2013): 3272–3291, accessed September 8, 2015, http://www.jci.org/articles/view/67674.

4.   R. J. Colman et al., "Caloric Restriction Delays Disease Onset and Mortality in Rhesus Monkeys," *Science* 325, no. 5937 (July 10, 2009): 201–204, doi:10.1126/science.1173635.

5.   Ibid.

6.   Bradley J. Willcox et al., "Caloric Restriction, the Traditional Okinawan Diet, and Healthy Aging," *Annals of the New*

York Academy of Sciences 1114 (2007): 434–455, doi:10.1196 /annals.1396.037.

7.   Ibid.

8.   R. L. Walford et al., "Physiologic Changes in Humans Subjected to Severe, Selective Calorie Restriction for Two Years in Biosphere 2: Health, Aging, and Toxicological Perspectives," *Journal of Toxicological Sciences* 52, 2 Supplement (December 1999): 61–65, http://www.ncbi.nlm.nih.gov/pubmed/10630592.

9.   James Rochon et al., "Design and Conduct of the CAL-ERIE Study: Comprehensive Assessment of the Long-Term Effects of Reducing Intake of Energy," *Journals of Gerontology, Series A, Biological Sciences and Medical Sciences* 66A, no. 1 (2011): 97–108, http://biomedgerontology.oxfordjournals.org/content/66A/1/97.

10.   A. V. Witte et al., "Caloric Restriction Improves Memory in Elderly Humans," *Proceedings of the National Academy of Sciences of the United States of America* 106, no. 4 (January 27, 2009): 1255–1260, doi:10.1073/pnas.0808587106.

11.   Michael Lefevre et al., "Caloric Restriction Alone and With Exercise Improves CVD Risk in Healthy Non-Obese Individuals," *Atherosclerosis* 203, no. 1 (March 2009): 206–213, doi:10.1016/j.atherosclerosis.2008.05.036.

12.   M. Meydani et al., "The Effect of Caloric Restriction and Glycemic Load on Measures of Oxidative Stress and Antioxidants in Humans: Results from the CALERIE Trial of Human Caloric Restriction," *The Journal of Nutrition Health and Aging* 15, no. 6 (June 2011): 456–460, http://www.ncbi.nlm.nih.gov/pubmed /21623467.

13.   L. K. Heilbronn et al., "Effect of 6-Month Calorie Restriction on Biomarkers of Longevity, Metabolic Adaptation, and Oxidative Stress in Overweight Individuals: A Randomized Controlled Trial," *Journal of the American Medical Association* 295, no. 13 (April 5, 2006): 1539–1548, http://www.ncbi.nlm.nih .gov/pubmed/16595757.

14.   A. E. Civitarese et al., "Calorie Restriction Increases Muscle Mitochondrial Biogenesis in Healthy Humans," *PLOS Medicine* 4, no. 3 (March 2007): e76, http://www.ncbi.nlm.nih .gov/pubmed/17341128.

15.   D. E. Larson-Meyer et al., "Effect of Calorie Restriction With or Without Exercise on Insulin Sensitivity, Beta-Cell

Function, Fat Cell Size, and Ectopic Lipid in Overweight Subjects," *Diabetes Care* 29, no. 6 (June 2006): 1337–1344, http://www.ncbi.nlm.nih.gov/pubmed/16732018.

CHAPTER 4
WHY FASTING WORKS

1.   "Benjamin Franklin Quotes," BrainyQuote, accessed September 4, 2015, http://www.brainyquote.com/quotes/quotes/b/benjaminfr379644.html.

2.   S. I. Rattan, "Hormesis in Aging," *Ageing Research Reviews* 7, no. 1 (January 2008): 63–78, http://www.ncbi.nlm.nih.gov/pubmed/17964227.

3.   Edward J. Masoro, "Role of Hormesis in Life Extension by Caloric Restriction," *Dose Response* 5, no 2 (2007): 163–173, http://www.ncbi.nlm.nih.gov/pmc/articles/PMC2477693/.

4.   Mattson, "Hormesis Defined."

5.   J. Viña et al., "Mechanism of Free Radical Production in Exhaustive Exercise in Humans and Rats; Role of Xanthine Oxidase and Protection by Allopurinol," *IUBMB Life* 49, no. 6 (June 2000): 539–544, http://www.ncbi.nlm.nih.gov/pubmed/11032249.

6.   Ibid.

7.   Rattan, "Hormesis in Aging."

8.   Ibid.

9.   This claim comes from two studies. The first is Masoro's "Role of Hormesis in Life Extension by Caloric Restriction" in endnote 3. The other is K. P. Keenan et al., "The Effects of Diet, Overfeeding and Moderate Dietary Restriction on Sprague-Dawley Rat Survival, Disease and Toxicology," *Journal of Nutrition* 127, supplement 5 (May 1997): 851S–856S, http://www.ncbi.nlm.nih.gov/pubmed/9164252.

10.   Jana Koubova and Leonard Guarente, "How Does Calorie Restriction Work?" *Genes & Development* 17 (2003): 313–321, http://genesdev.cshlp.org/content/17/3/313.full.

11.   A. Munck, P. M. Guyre, and N. J. Holbrook, "Physiological Functions of Glucocorticoids in Stress and Their Relation to Pharmacological Actions," *Endocrine Reviews* 5, no. 1 (Winter 1984): 25–44, http://www.ncbi.nlm.nih.gov/pubmed/6368214.

12.   A. G. Schwartz and L. L. Pashko, "Cancer Prevention With Dehydroepiandrosterone and Non-Androgenic Structural Analogs," *Journal of Cellular Biochemistry Supplement* 22 (1995): 210–217, http://www.ncbi.nlm.nih.gov/pubmed/8538200.

13.   R. S. Sohal and R. Weindruch, "Oxidative Stress, Caloric Restriction, and Aging," *Science* 273, no. 5271 (July 5, 1996): 59–63, http://www.ncbi.nlm.nih.gov/pubmed/8658196.

14.   Borut Poljsak, "Strategies for Reducing or Preventing the Generation of Oxidative Stress," *Oxidative Medicine and Cellular Longevity* 2011 (2011), http://www.ncbi.nlm.nih.gov/pubmed/22191011.

15.   B. N. Ames, "Micronutrient Deficiencies. A Major Cause of DNA Damage," *Annals of the New York Academy of Sciences* 889 (1999): 87–106, http://www.ncbi.nlm.nih.gov/pubmed/10668486.

16.   Borut Poljsak, Dušan Šuput, and Irina Milisav, "Achieving the Balance Between ROS and Antioxidants: When to Use the Synthetic Antioxidants," *Oxidative Medicine and Cellular Longevity* 2013 (2013): 956792, http://www.ncbi.nlm.nih.gov/pmc/articles/PMC3657405/.

17.   Poljsak, "Strategies for Reducing or Preventing the Generation of Oxidative Stress."

18.   Ibid.; Poljsak, Šuput, and Milisav "Achieving the Balance Between ROS and Antioxidants: When to Use the Synthetic Antioxidants."

19.   Poljsak, "Strategies for Reducing or Preventing the Generation of Oxidative Stress."

20.   X. Qiu et al., "Calorie Restriction Reduces Oxidative Stress by SIRT3-Mediated SOD2 Activation," *Cell Metabolism* 12, no. 6 (December 2010): 662–667, http://www.ncbi.nlm.nih.gov/pubmed/21109198.

21.   Mattson, "Hormesis Defined."

22.   Poljsak, "Strategies for Reducing or Preventing the Generation of Oxidative Stress."

CHAPTER 5
PREVENTING DIABETES

1.   Don Colbert, *Reversing Diabetes* (Lake Mary, FL: Siloam, 2012), 2.

2.   These figures come from the Radiological Society of North America, "Restricted Calorie Diet Improves Heart Function in Obese Patients With Diabetes," November 28, 2011, accessed September 8, 2015, http://www2.rsna.org/timssnet /media/pressreleases/pr_target.cfm?id=560; S. Hammar et al., "Prolonged Caloric Restriction in Obese Patients With Type 2 Diabetes Mellitus Decreases Myocardial Triglyceride Content and Improves Myocardial Function," *Journal of American College of Cardiology* 52, no. 12 (September 16, 2008): 1006–1012, http:// www.ncbi.nlm.nih.gov/pubmed/18786482.

3.   "National Diabetes Statistics Report, 2014," Centers for Disease Control and Prevention, accessed September 7, 2015, http://www.cdc.gov/diabetes/pubs/statsreport14/national-diabetes -report-web.pdf.

4.   Larson-Meyer et al., "Effect of Calorie Restriction With or Without Exercise on Insulin Sensitivity, Beta-Cell Function, Fat Cell Size, and Ectopic Lipid in Overweight Subjects."

5.   S. Polovina and D. Micić, "The Influence of Diet With Reduction in Calorie Intake on Metabolic Syndrome Parameters in Obese Subjects With Impaired Glucose Tolerance," *Medicinski Pregled* 63, no. 7–8 (July–August 2010): 465–469, http://www.ncbi .nlm.nih.gov/pubmed/21446131.

6.   Ibid.

7.   M. A. Lane, D. K. Ingram, and G. S. Roth, "Calorie Restriction in Nonhuman Primates: Effects on Diabetes and Cardiovascular Disease Risk," *Journal of Toxicological Sciences* 52, 2 supplement (December 1999): 41–48, http://www.ncbi.nlm.nih .gov/pubmed/10630589.

8.   A. R. Barnosky et al., "Intermittent Fasting vs Daily Calorie Restriction for Type 2 Diabetes Prevention: A Review of Human Findings," *Translational Research* 164, no. 4 (October 2014): 302–311, http://www.ncbi.nlm.nih.gov/pubmed/24993615.

9.   Ibid.

10.   Ibid.

11.   J. Merino et al., "Body Weight Loss by Very-Low -Calorie Diet Program Improves Small Artery Reactive Hyperemia in Severely Obese Patients," *Obesity Surgery* 23, no. 1 (January 2013): 17–23, http://www.ncbi.nlm.nih.gov/pubmed /22918551; "UK Prospective Diabetes Study 7: Response of Fasting

Plasma Glucose to Diet Therapy in Newly Presenting Type II Diabetic Patients," UKPDS Group, *Metabolism* 39, no. 9 (September 1990): 905–912, http://www.ncbi.nlm.nih.gov/pubmed/2392060.

12.   Ibid.

13.   "UK Prospective Diabetes Study 7: Response of Fasting Plasma Glucose to Diet Therapy in Newly Presenting Type II Diabetic Patients," UKPDS Group.

14.   Ilaria Malandrucco et al., "Very-Low-Calorie Diet: A Quick Therapeutic Tool to Improve β Cell Function in Morbidly Obese Patients With Type 2 Diabetes," *American Journal of Clinical Nutrition* 95, no. 3 (March 2012): 609–613, http://ajcn.nutrition.org/content/95/3/609.long#ref-1.

15.   Ibid.

CHAPTER 6
REDUCING CANCER RISKS

1.   Valter D. Longo and Luigi Fontana, "Calorie Restriction and Cancer Prevention: Metabolic and Molecular Mechanisms," *Trends in Pharmacological Sciences* 31, no. 2 (February 2010): 89–98, http://www.ncbi.nlm.nih.gov/pmc/articles/PMC2829867/.

2.   National Cancer Institute, NCI Fact Sheets, "Cancer Statistics," accessed September 7, 2015, http://www.cancer.gov/about-cancer/what-is-cancer/statistics.

3.   Longo and Fontana, "Calorie Restriction and Cancer Prevention: Metabolic and Molecular Mechanisms."

4.   D. Kritchevsky, "Caloric Restriction and Cancer," *Journal of Nutritional Science and Vitaminology (Tokyo)* 47, no. 1 (February 2001): 13–19, http://www.ncbi.nlm.nih.gov/pubmed/11349885.

5.   D. Albanes, "Caloric Intake, Body Weight, and Cancer: A Review," *Nutrition and Cancer* 9, no. 4 (1987): 199–217, http://www.ncbi.nlm.nih.gov/pubmed/3299283.

6.   Ibid.

7.   Colman et al., "Caloric Restriction Delays Disease Onset and Mortality in Rhesus Monkeys."

8.   Fernando M. Safdie et al., "Fasting and Cancer Treatment in Humans: A Case Series Report," *Aging* (Albany NY) 1,

no. 12 (December 2009): 988–1007, http://www.ncbi.nlm.nih.gov/pmc/articles/PMC2815756/.

9.   J. W. Lee et al., "Protein Kinase A-Alpha Directly Phosphorylates FoxO1 in Vascular Endothelial Cells to Regulate Expression of Vascular Cellular Adhesion Molecule-1 mRNA," *The Journal of Biological Chemistry* 286, no. 8 (February 25, 2011): 6423–6432, doi:10.1074/jbc.M110.180661.

10.   C. W. Cheng et al., "Prolonged Fasting Reduces IGF-1/PKA to Promote Hematopoietic-Stem-Cell-Based Regeneration and Reverse Immunosuppression," *Cell Stem Cell* 14, no. 6 (June 5, 2014): 810–823, doi:10.1016/j.stem.2014.04.014.

11.   Lee Changhan et al., "Fasting Cycles Retard Growth of Tumors and Sensitize a Range of Cancer Cell Types to Chemotherapy," *Science Translation Medicine* 4, no. 124 (March 7, 2012): 124ra27, doi:10.1126/scitranslmed.3003293.

12.   Ibid.

13.   Olga P. Rogozina et al., "Effect of Chronic and Intermittent Calorie Restriction on Serum Adiponectin and Leptin and Mammary Tumorigenesis," *Cancer Prevention Research (Philadelphia)* 4, no. 4 (April 2011): 568–581, doi:10.1158/1940-6207.CAPR-10-0140.

14.   C. Galet et al., "Effects of Calorie Restriction and IGF-1 Receptor Blockade on the Progression of 22Rv1 Prostate Cancer Xenografts," *International Journal of Molecular Sciences* 14, no. 7 (July 3, 2013): 13782–95, doi:10.3390/ijms140713782.

CHAPTER 7
CARE FOR YOUR HEART

1.   "Abraham Lincoln Quotes," Brainy Quote, http://www.brainyquote.com/quotes/quotes/a/abrahamlin137180.html.

2.   Colman et al., "Caloric Restriction Delays Disease Onset and Mortality in Rhesus Monkeys."

3.   J. A. Mattison et al., "Impact of Caloric Restriction on Health and Survival in Rhesus Monkeys From the NIA Study," *Nature* 489, no. 7415 (September 13, 2012): 318–321, doi:10.1038/nature11432.

4.   Lefevre et al., "Caloric Restriction Alone and With Exercise Improves CVD Risk in Healthy Non-Obese Individuals."

5.   "What Is Atherosclerosis?", National Heart, Lung, and Blood Institute, accessed November 10, 2015, http://www.nhlbi .nih.gov/health/health-topics/topics/atherosclerosis.

6.   "What Is Atherosclerosis?", WebMD, accessed November 10, 2015, http://www.webmd.com/heart-disease/what-is -atherosclerosis.

7.   "Heart Disease and Stroke Statistics—At-a-Glance," The American Heart Association and the American Stroke Association, 2015, http://www.heart.org/idc/groups/ahamah-public /@wcm/@sop/@smd/documents/downloadable/ucm_470704.pdf.

8.   "What Is Atherosclerosis?" National Heart, Lung, and Blood Institute and WebMD,

9.   C. W. Bales and W. E. Kraus, "Caloric Restriction: Implications for Human Cardiometabolic Health," *Journal of Cardiopulmonary Rehabilitation and Prevention* 33, no. 4 (2013): 201–208, http://www.ncbi.nlm.nih.gov/pubmed/23748374.

CHAPTER 8
BOOST YOUR BRAIN

1.   "Quote by Plato," Quotery.com, accessed September 8, 2015, http://www.quotery.com/quotes/i-fast-for-greater-physical -and-mental-efficiency/.

2.   Mark Mattson, "Why Fasting Bolsters Brain Power," TEDx Talk, 2014, accessed September 7, 2015, http://tedxtalks.ted .com/video/Why-Fasting-Bolsters-Brain-Powe.

3.   Marwan A. Maalouf, Jong M. Rho, and Mark P. Mattson, "The Neuroprotective Properties of Calorie Restriction, the Ketogenic Diet, and Ketone Bodies," *Brain Research Reviews* 59, no. 2 (2009): 293–315, doi:10.1016/j.brainresrev.2008.09.002.

4.   Devin K. Binder and Helen E. Scharfman, "Brain-Derived Neurotrophic Factor," *Growth Factors* 22, no. 3 (September 2004): 123–131, http://www.ncbi.nlm.nih.gov/pmc /articles/PMC2504526/pdf/nihms58796.pdf.

5.   Tytus Murphy, Gisele Pereira Dias, and Sandrine Thuret, "Effects of Diet on Brain Plasticity in Animal and Human Studies: Mind the Gap," *Neural Plasticity* 2014 (2014): 563160, doi:10.1155/2014/563160.

6. John Gabrieli, "The Brain," MIT OpenCourseware, accessed September 8, 2015, http://ocw.mit.edu/courses/brain-and -cognitive-sciences/9-00sc-introduction-to-psychology-fall-2011 /brain-i/MIT9_00SCF11_lec03_brain1.pdf.

7. N. Mizushima et al., "Autophagy Fights Disease Through Cellular Self-Digestion," *Nature* 451, no. 7182 (February 28, 2008): 1069–1075, doi:10.1038/nature06639.

8. Ibid.

9. Public image of a neuron retrieved from John Gabrieli, "The Brain," MIT, http://ocw.mit.edu/courses/brain-and-cognitive -sciences/9-00sc-introduction-to-psychology-fall-2011/brain-i /MIT9_00SCF11_lec03_brain1.pdf. Public domain: http://ocw.mit .edu/terms/.

10. Information from Mizushima et al., "Autophagy Fights Disease Through Cellular Self-Digestion"; Jin H. Son et al., "Neuronal Autophagy and Neurodegenerative Diseases," *Experimental & Molecular Medicine* 44 (2012): 89–98, doi:10.3858/emm.2012 .44.2.031.

11. Mehrdad Alirezaei et al., "Short-Term Fasting Induces Profound Neuronal Autophagy," *Autophagy* 6, no. 6 (August 2010): 702–710, doi:10.4161/auto.6.6.12376.

12. Ibid.

13. Maalouf, Rho, and Mattson, "The Neuroprotective Properties of Calorie Restriction, the Ketogenic Diet, and Ketone Bodies."

14. Ibid.

15. Information comes from Maalouf, Rho, and Mattson, "The Neuroprotective Properties of Calorie Restriction, the Ketogenic Diet, and Ketone Bodies." See also A. Lutas and G. Yellen, "The Ketogenic Diet: Metabolic Influences on Brain Excitability and Epilepsy," *Trends in Neurosciences* 36, no. 1 (January 2013): 32–40. doi:10.1016/j.tins.2012.11.005.

16. Mark P. Mattson and Tim Magnus, "Aging and Neuronal Vulnerability," *Nature Reviews Neuroscience* 7, no. 4 (2006): 278–294, doi:10.1038/nrn1886.

17. Marwan Maalouf et al., "Ketones Inhibit Mitochondrial Production of Reactive Oxygen Species Production Following Glutamate Excitotoxicity by Increasing NADH Oxidation,"

Neuroscience 145, no. 1 (March 2, 2007): 256–264, doi:10.1016/j.neuroscience.2006.11.065.

18. Maalouf, Rho, and Mattson, "The Neuroprotective Properties of Calorie Restriction, the Ketogenic Diet, and Ketone Bodies."

19. "Depression," Centers for Disease Control and Prevention, accessed September 6, 2015, http://www.cdc.gov/nchs/fastats/depression.htm.

20. "Current Depression Among Adults, United States, 2006 and 2008," Morbidity and Mortality Weekly Report (MMWR), Centers for Disease Control and Prevention, accessed November 2, 2015, http://www.ncbi.nlm.nih.gov/pubmed/20881934.

21. "Depression," Centers for Disease Control and Prevention.

22. A. Michalsen et al., "Prolonged Fasting in Patients With Chronic Pain Syndromes Leads to Late Mood-Enhancement Not Related to Weight Loss and Fasting-Induced Leptin Depletion," *Nutritional Neuroscience* 9, no. 5–6 (October–December 2006): 195–200, http://www.ncbi.nlm.nih.gov/pubmed/17263085.

23. Ibid.

24. Guillaume Fond et al., "Fasting in Mood Disorders: Neurobiology and Effectiveness. A Review of the Literature," *Psychiatry Research* 209, no. 3 (October 30, 2013): 253–258, doi:10.1016/j.psychres.2012.12.018.

25. N. I. Teng et al., "Efficacy of Fasting Calorie Restriction on Quality of Life Among Aging Men," *Physiology & Behavior* 104, no. 5 (October 24, 2011): 1059–1064, doi:10.1016/j.physbeh.2011.07.007.

26. Yun Li et al., "TrkB Regulates Hippocampal Neurogenesis and Governs Sensitivity to Antidepressive Treatment," *Neuron* 59, no. 3 (August 14, 2008): 399–412, doi:10.1016/j.neuron.2008.06.023.

27. Heath D. Schmidt and Ronald S. Duman, "Peripheral BDNF Produces Antidepressant-Like Effects in Cellular and Behavioral Models," *Neuropsychopharmacology* 35, no. 12 (November 2010): 2378–2391, doi:10.1038/npp.2010.114.

28. Ibid.

29. Ángela Fontán-Lozano et al., "Molecular Bases of Caloric Restriction Regulation of Neuronal Synaptic Plasticity,"

Molecular Neurobiology 38, no. 2 (October 2008): 167–177, doi:10.1007/s12035-008-8040-1.

30.   Andrew J. Brown, "Low-Carb Diets, Fasting and Euphoria: Is There a Link between Ketosis and Gamma -Hydroxybutyrate (GHB)?" *Medical Hypotheses* 68, no. 2 (2007): 268–271, http://www.ncbi.nlm.nih.gov/pubmed/17011713.

31.   Fond et al., "Fasting in Mood Disorders: Neurobiology and Effectiveness. A Review of the Literature."

32.   D. K. Ingram et al., "Dietary Restriction Benefits Learning and Motor Performance of Aged Mice," *Journals of Gerontology* 42, no. 1 (January 1987): 78–81, http://www.ncbi.nlm .nih.gov/pubmed/3794202.

33.   Witte et al., "Caloric Restriction Improves Memory in Elderly Humans."

34.   Ibid.

35.   "2015 Alzheimer's Disease Facts and Figures," Alzheimer's Association, accessed November 10, 2015, http://www.alz.org /facts/overview.asp.

36.   Ibid.

37.   Murphy, Dias, and Thuret, "Effects of Diet on Brain Plasticity in Animal and Human Studies: Mind the Gap."

38.   "2015 Alzheimer's Disease Facts and Figures," Alzheimer's Association

39.   Pu Wu et al., "Calorie Restriction Ameliorates Neurode-generative Phenotypes in Forebrain-Specific Presenilin-1 and Pre-senilin-2 Double Knockout Mice," *Neurobiology of Aging* 29, no. 10 (October 2008): 1502–1511, http://www.sciencedirect.com /science/article/pii/S0197458007001376.

40.   Murphy, Dias, and Thuret, "Effects of Diet on Brain Plasticity in Animal and Human Studies: Mind the Gap."

41.   M. Kivipelto et al., "Obesity and Vascular Risk Factors at Midlife and the Risk of Dementia and Alzheimer Disease," *Archives of Neurology* 62, no. 10 (October 2005): 1556–1560, http://www.ncbi.nlm.nih.gov/pubmed/16216938.

42.   Ibid.

43.   Maalouf, Rho, and Mattson, "The Neuroprotective Properties of Calorie Restriction, the Ketogenic Diet, and Ketone Bodies"; Jose A. Luchsinger, Ming-Xing Tang, Steven Shea, and Richard Mayeux, "Caloric Intake and the Risk of Alzheimer

Disease," *JAMA Neurology* 59, no. 8 (2002):1258–1263, http://archneur.jaman etwork.com/article.aspx?articleid=782575.

44. "NINDS Stroke Information Page," National Institute of Neurological Disorders and Stroke, accessed September 6, 2015, http://www.ninds.nih.gov/disorders/stroke/stroke.htm.

45. "Heart Disease and Stroke Statistics—At-a-Glance," The American Heart Association and the American Stroke Association.

46. Silvia Manzanero et al., "Calorie Restriction and Stroke," *Experimental & Translational Stroke Medicine* 3 (2011): 8, http://www.ncbi.nlm.nih.gov/pmc/articles/PMC3179731/.

47. O. Lindvall et al., "Differential Regulation of mRNAs for Nerve Growth Factor, Brain-Derived Neurotrophic Factor, and Neurotrophin 3 in the Adult Rat Brain Following Cerebral Ischemia and Hypoglycemic Coma," *Proceedings for the National Academy of Sciences USA* 89, no. 2 (January 15, 1992): 648–652, http://www.ncbi.nlm.nih.gov/pmc/articles/PMC48296/.

CHAPTER 9
HEALTH BENEFITS OF CHRISTIAN FASTING

1. Early Church Fathers, Twitter post, March 6, 2014, 1:30 p.m., accessed September 8, 2015, https://twitter.com/early_church/status/441642012798763008.

2. Richard J. Bloomer et al., "Effect of a 21 Day Daniel Fast on Metabolic and Cardiovascular Disease Risk Factors in Men and Women," *Lipids in Health and Disease* 9 (2010): 94, doi:10.1186/1476-511X-9-94.

3. Ibid.

4. Richard J. Bloomer et al., "A 21 Day Daniel Fast Improves Selected Biomarkers of Antioxidant Status and Oxidative Stress in Men and Women," *Nutrition & Metabolism* 8 (2011): 17, doi:10.1186/1743-7075-8-17.

5. "Good vs. Bad Cholesterol," American Heart Association, January 12, 2015, accessed September 6, 2015, http://www.heart.org/HEARTORG/Conditions/Cholesterol/AboutCholesterol/Good-vs-Bad-Cholesterol_UCM_305561_Article.jsp.

6. Rick J. Alleman et al., "Both a Traditional and Modified Daniel Fast Improve the Cardio-Metabolic Profile in Men

and Women," *Lipids in Health and Disease* 12 (2013): 114, doi:10.1186/1476-511X-12-114.

7.   John F. Trepanowski and Richard J. Bloomer, "The Impact of Religious Fasting on Human Health," *Nutrition Journal* 9 (2010): 57, doi:10.1186/1475-2891-9-57.

CHAPTER 10
FASTING FOR TOTAL WELL-BEING

1.   D. A. Williamson et al., "Is Caloric Restriction Associated With Development of Eating-Disorder Symptoms? Results from the CALERIE trial," *Health Psychology* 27, 1 Supplement (January 2008): S32–42, doi:10.1037/0278-6133.27.1.S32.

2.   Ibid.

CHAPTER 11
DIFFERENT PLANS

1.   "22 Ole Hallesby Quotes," Christian Quotes, accessed September 6, 2015, http://www.christianquotes.info/quotes-by -author/ole-hallesby-quotes/.

2.   "Andrew Bonar on Fasting," Christian Quotes, accessed September 6, 2015, http://christian-quotes.ochristian.com /christian-quotes_ochristian.cgi?find=Christian-quotes-by -Andrew+Bonar-on-Fasting.

CHAPTER 12
FASTING FOR LIFE

1.   Thomas Ryan, *The Sacred Art of Fasting: Preparing to Practice* (Woodstock, VT: Skylight Paths Publishing, 2006), 163–164.

2.   "William Feather Quotes," BrainyQuote, accessed September 6, 2015, http://www.brainyquote.com/quotes/authors/w /william_feather.html.

3.   Eugene H. Peterson, *The Pastor: A Memoir* (San Francisco: Harper One, 2010), 240.

CHAPTER 13
FASTING AND SPIRITUAL RENEWAL

1.   "Fasting Quotes: Early Church Fathers," Fasting for God, August 2, 2011, accessed September 6, 2015, http://fastingforgod .org/?tag=st-augustine.
2.   "Wesley L. Duewel Quotes," ChristianQuotes.com, accessed September 6, 2015, http://christian-quotes.ochristian .com/Wesley-L.-Duewel-Quotes/.
3.   Denise Levertov, "Overland to the Islands," 1958, popularized by Eugene Peterson's *The Pastor: A Memoir*.

CHAPTER 16
PRAYING THE SCRIPTURES

1.   Bill Thrasher, *A Journey to Victorious Praying* (Chicago: Moody Publishers, 2003), 143.
2.   Carl Rogers, *On Becoming a Person: A Therapist's View of Psychotherapy*, quoted at GoodReads, "Carl Rogers Quotes," accessed September 6, 2015, http://www.goodreads.com/author /quotes/102062.Carl_R_Rogers.

CHAPTER 17
FASTING AND FORGIVENESS

1.   Deacon Keith Fournier, "St. Peter Chrysologus: Prayer Knocks, Fasting Obtains, Mercy Receives," accessed September 6, 2015, http://www.beliefnet.com/columnists/bread_on_the_trail /2011/03/st-peter-chrysologus-prayer-knocks-fasting-obtains -mercy-receives.html.
2.   "Divorce Rates by State: 1990, 1995, and 1999–2011, Centers for Disease Control and Prevention, accessed September 6, 2015, http://www.cdc.gov/nchs/data/dvs/divorce_rates_90_95_99 -11.pdf.
3.   Jennifer Glass, "Red States, Blue States, and Divorce: Understanding the Impact of Conservative Protestantism on Regional Variation in Divorce Rates," *American Journal of Sociology*, 119, no. 4 (January 2014):1002-1046, http://www.ncbi.nlm .nih.gov/pubmed/25032268.

4.   "William Blake Quotes," BrainyQuote, accessed September 6, 2015, http://www.brainyquote.com/quotes/quotes/w/williambla101447.html.

5.   "Lewis B. Smedes Quotes," BrainyQuote, accessed September 6, 2015, http://www.brainyquote.com/quotes/quotes/l/lewisbsme135524.html.

Chapter 18
Prayer Walks

1.   As quoted in "Health Epigrams," *Young Men*, 41, no. 1 (October 1915), 4.

2.   "Friedrich Nietzsche Quotes," BrainyQuote, accessed September 7, 2015, http://www.brainyquote.com/quotes/quotes/f/friedrichn162010.html.

3.   "The Benefits of Walking," American Heart Association, accessed September 7, 2015, http://www.startwalkingnow.org/whystart_benefits_walking.jsp.

4.   Richard Weil, "Walking," MedicineNet.com, April 17, 2015, accessed September 7, 2015, http://www.medicinenet.com/walking/article.htm#what_are_the_top_10_reasons_to_walk; Javed Butler, "Primary Prevention of Heart Failure," *ISRN Cardiology* 2012 (2012), doi:10.5402/2012/982417.

5.   National Diabetes Information Clearinghouse, "Diabetes Prevention Program," National Institute of Diabetes and Digestive and Kidney Diseases, October 2008, accessed September 7, 2015, http://www.niddk.nih.gov/about-niddk/research-areas/diabetes/diabetes-prevention-program-dpp/Pages/default.aspx; W. C. Knowler et al., "Reduction in the Incidence of Type 2 Diabetes With Lifestyle Intervention or Metformin," *New England Journal of Medicine* 346, no. 6 (February 7, 2002): 393–403, http://www.ncbi.nlm.nih.gov/pubmed/11832527.

6.   Ibid.

7.   Weil, "Walking"; Butler, "Primary Prevention of Heart Failure."

8.   Weil, "Walking."

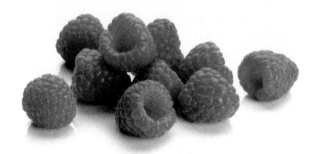

A Healthy Life—
body, mind, and spirit—
IS PART OF GOD'S PURPOSE FOR YOU!

Siloam brings you books, e-books, and other media from trusted authors on today's most important health topics. Check out the following links for more books from specialists such as *New York Times* best-selling author Dr. Don Colbert and get on the road to great health.

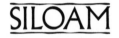

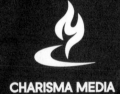